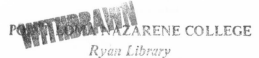

# HUMAN LONGEVITY

# HUMAN
# LONGEVITY

DAVID W. E. SMITH

Professor, Department of Pathology and Buehler Center on Aging
Northwestern University Medical School
Chicago, Illinois

*New York    Oxford*
OXFORD UNIVERSITY PRESS
*1993*

Oxford University Press

Oxford   New York   Toronto
Delhi   Bombay   Calcutta   Madras   Karachi
Kuala Lumpur   Singapore   Hong Kong   Tokyo
Nairobi   Dar es Salaam   Cape Town
Melbourne   Auckland   Madrid

and associated companies in
Berlin   Ibadan

Library of Congress Cataloging-in-Publication Data
Smith, David W. E.
Human longevity / David W.E. Smith.
p.   cm.
Includes bibliographical references and index.
ISBN 0-19-508313-X
1. Longevity.   I. Title.
[DNLM:   1. Longevity—genetics.   WT 104 S645h]
   QP85.S497   1993
   612.6′8—dc20
   DNLM/DLC
   for Library of Congress          92-49136

9 8 7 6 5 4 3 2 1

Printed in the United States of America
on acid-free paper

To Diane

# Preface

This volume is offered as an original treatment on the subject of human longevity. The approach is multidisciplinary, and the main contributing disciplines are:

1. *Life Sciences.* The biological changes leading to human mortality occur on several levels, including the molecular, the cellaular, the organ and system, and the integrated organism. There are genetic determinants of life span, and the long human life span has been subject to evolution.
2. *Medicine and Pathology.* Most human life is terminated by recognizable causes, and an understanding of the common causes of mortality goes beyond an appreciation of the biology. During the last century, the diseases that cause death have changed, and the diseases of mortality in developed countries are now diseases of later life. The epidemiology of human mortality must be considered in the context of the epidemiology and pathogenesis of these diseases. As the mean human life span grows even longer, the causes of death may continue to change.
3. *Social Sciences.* Demographers describe the length of human life in various situations, and there is much diversity. The risks and risk factors of mortality are based on human behavior and on conditions in human societies, but not all of the demographic diversity in longevity that is observed can be explained on the basis of risks and risk factors recognized today.

The uniqueness and the strength of this book are the presentation of extensive information from these disciplines and the interdisciplinary synthesis of ideas and conclusions about human longevity.

The book's focus is sharpened by the exclusion of two related subjects found in other books, that would appear to be similar. (1) One of these is aging. Senescence is defined as the condition in which the rate of mortality increases with age. Senescent changes cause disability and precede mortality in ways that are often obvious. There is much individual variation in senescent changes, and no fixed schedule. The study of aging examines many phenomena that have no certain relationship to mortality. Mortality has the added advantage of being an all or none condition, whereas aspects of aging are relative. (2) The other exclusion is a limitation of this book to the human species. Although some attention is given to a comparison of human life spans with those of other living things, and although it is recognized that humans have some characteristics in common with other living things, an important theme of this book is that much about human longevity is unique. Not only is the maximum human life span about twice that of the next most longevous mammal, but the common causes of human death are different from any other animal. No other animal has been studied as exhaustively as the human species. Treatments of longevity emphasizing, for example, fruit flies or rodents must offer different coverage than this book.

This book is written for the professional in one of the disciplines with an interest in longevity, who wants to review what the other disciplines have to offer, and for other readers who want a balanced and comprehensive treatment of this important subject. The level of sophistication and the vocabulary are selected to serve these audiences, with the understanding that both professionals and other readers probably know something about one or more of the disciplines related to longevity but that each reader is seeking coverage on a broader basis.

Each chapter can stand alone as a review of its topic, but a value is intended in starting with Chapter 1 and reading through the book. There is a logic to the organization based on questions that arise, as described briefly at the end of Chapter 1.

Almost every page of this volume could be expanded into a book, and many such books have been written by other authors, although human longevity is usually not the focus. Some readers may need to consult basic textbooks in different disciplines for explanations, for example, of classic genetics, sex hormones, life tables, and blood clotting. Alternatively, readers with some expertise in one of the disciplines will find sections of the book that they need not read. I hope this volume occupies a middle ground between too much explanation of well-established basic concepts and so little explanation that the treatment of longevity seems glib or obscure.

Most of the tables and figures present demographic and epidemiological data. They are usually only a sampling, carefully chosen, of much more comprehensive data in the sources cited. Often data from multiple sources are combined or calculations have been done resulting in new data. The tables offered do not duplicate tables published elsewhere. The intention is that enough data are included in the tables and figures to support and exemplify the statements made. Readers using this as a reference book will find values that can be cited. The data are from the years indicated and are up-to-date as of the time of writing, but some sources are updated regularly, with new editions. The interested reader will find current versions of *Vital Statistics of the United States* published by the National Center for Health Statistics and the *Demographic Yearbook* published by the United Nations to be rich sources of information from which many additional tables and figures could be composed.

Shorter tables are integrated into the text. In general they illustrate limited points and are cited in one place in the text. Longer tables, which are usually cited in multiple places, and which tend to break up the text, are located in the Appendix at the back of the book.

Nearly 400 references are cited and are listed at the end of the book. The reference list could easily be ten or even a hundred times longer if an effort had been made to provide full documentation of every statement from primary sources. Well-established information, available in basic textbooks, is not cited. Most of the citations are from the research literature. When possible, summaries, such as review papers and book chapters, are cited to support statements. The result is that many primary research papers that were seminal in the development of ideas presented in this volume are not cited here, although they are cited in the bibliographies of the chapters and review papers. Primary research papers are cited, when they are recent, when they have not been covered by reviews, or when they themselves contain substantial reviews of the literature.

Having made the above case for the originality of this volume, I must acknowledge several publications by others that played important roles in the development and structure of this book. They include those of Cutler, 1975; Finch, 1990; Hayflick, 1987; Hazzard, 1986; Kirkwood, 1985; Nathanson, 1984; and Olshansky, 1988. I also received much help from colleagues who discussed ideas and read sections of the manuscript. The reference staff of the Medical Library of Northwestern University was generous in finding references and in obtaining volumes from other libraries. The computer graphics used as figures were kindly provided by Dr. Jayme Borensztajn-Brentan, Professor of Pathology at Northwestern University. Finally, I express my gratitude to Ms. Lowella Rivero of Northwestern University who typed the manuscript with much skill and more than a little artistry and saw it through many changes.

*Chicago*                                                                                          D. S.
*March 1993*

# Contents

# HUMAN LONGEVITY

# Mortality:
# Survival and Longevity

there is a great difference between going off in warm blood like Romeo and making one's
exit like a frog in a frost.

JOHN KEATS (1795–1821)
Letter to Fanny Brawne, 1820 (Gittings, 1968)

Human life is long today. The mean life expectancy at birth in the United States
is 75 years for both sexes, and many individuals live much longer than that.
There are two and a half million people 85 years old and over and about 30,000
people 100 years old and over in the United States today, and these numbers will
most certainly increase in the foreseeable future as people already living reach
advanced ages. Moreover, there are reasons to expect mean life expectancies to
become even greater. Someone returning from the early years of this century
would be surprised at the large numbers of elderly people and the paucity of
orphans (Blythe, 1969).

No doubt many readers are glad that human longevity is so long today and
look forward to rich elderly lives. At the same time it is widely recognized that
we live in an "aging society," and the increasing numbers of elderly people
present problems for everyone. This book does not propose solutions to the
problems, and it is not its purpose to provide the reader a prescription for
longevity. It does present the dimensions of human longevity in the past, present,
and future, discuss what has happened to change human longevity so much, and
explore the determinants of the human life span.

Chapter 1 is devoted largely to human longevity as it has varied over time and
place—the history and current demographics of longevity. The chapter begins
with definitions and a discussion of terms that embody concepts and will appear
frequently in this volume.

## Concepts and Definitions

### *Mortality Rates*

The term *mortality rate* is used often in this book. It refers to the number of
individuals dying in a population of a fixed number, usually 100,000, per unit of
time, usually one year for humans. The population may be of any desired
characteristic. In this volume, for example, mortality rates are described for
populations based on nation or political subdivision of residence, on gender, and
on race. Mortality rates are described for people of all ages and for people falling
into narrow age ranges (age-specific motality rates). The age structure of populations has a great effect on mortality rates because mortality usually increases with
age. Sometimes it is useful to compare mortality rates although the age structures
of populations differ greatly. Age adjustment permits the comparison of populations after corrections for age structure. The *age-adjusted mortality rate* is commonly made to the age structure of the U.S. population in 1940. In text and in
tables, mortality rates are clearly identified if they are age adjusted.

### *Life Span/Survival/Life Expectancy/Longevity*

The terms life span, survival, life expectancy, and longevity, which have multiple
usages, are used frequently and quite specifically in this volume, and are worth
discussing at the beginning.

   *Life span* means the time spent living by any individual of any species. It may
be long or short relative to the life spans of other individuals of the species or of
individuals of other species. It is possible to determine an average life span when
much is known about a population of individuals with some similar characteristics. The *maximum species life span* can be determined when the life spans of
large numbers of individuals living under favorable conditions are known. It is
the life span of the longest lived individual for which credible records exist, or
perhaps the life span of the longest lived percentile or decile. This figure is based
on outlyers.

   The word *survival* may apply to individuals, but the term *life span* is preferred
here. *Survival* is used chiefly as a determination made from survival curves.
These curves (e.g., Figs. 1-1, 1-2, and 1-3) describe the numbers or percentages
of a cohort remaining after the passage of measured amounts of time or at
specific ages. Ideally, a survival curve begins at the time of birth of the cohort
with 100 percent surviving and ends with the death of the last member of the
cohort. Data used in constructing survival curves can be used in constructing life
tables and in determining the mean age of survival of a population. The term
survival is also occasionally used to describe life that is sustained with difficulty

under adverse conditions. Survivors are individuals that have survived the adverse conditions longer than might have been expected.

The term *life expectancy* refers to the amount of life remaining. It is a value derived from life tables, which are based on the survival of a population. Life tables convert the multiple specific death rates for each age group in a population into the number of deaths in each interval per 100,000 of population (Dublin, 1922). It is, therefore, more appropriate to refer to a *mean life expectancy*. The mean life expectancy at any particular age can be determined. Most commonly, mean life expectancy at birth is described. Life expectancies are useful in comparing stable populations, but it must be recognized that the life spans of those who have recently died are used to calculate the life expectancies of those who are still living, including those who have just been born. At times when life spans are changing rapidly, life expectancies have little predictive value for events likely to occur in the distant future. Life expectancies that are often described in this volume are subject to these limitations.

The word *longevity*, which appears in the title of this book, is sometimes used interchangeably with life span, but not in this volume. Here, it is used as suggested by its Latin root and its common first definition to mean long life—a duration of life that approaches the maximum species life span. It is a word that has meaning at several levels. There are individuals displaying longevity. Most individuals in economically developed populations display longevity, and one can refer to the longevity of such populations including national populations. The terms maximum species life span and maximum species longevity are used interchangeably, especially in reference to humans.


## Animal Survival

Most living things die, although there are exceptions in the form of some one-celled organisms (bacteria and haploid protozoa), plants, and invertebrates that can reproduce indefinitely by the process of cell division (Smith-Sonneborn, 1987; Finch, 1990).

Considering mortal species, humans have a greater maximum life span than any other warm-blooded animal. Although the case will be made that much about human longevity is unique, there is something to be learned from comparing human longevity with the survival of other species. Among animals maximum life spans vary by a factor of about $10^4$, although all living things are composed of similar, but not identical, proteins and nucleic acids, and cells of all kinds require similar, but not identical, environments. Among mammals, maximum life spans vary by a factor of more than 100, with some insectivores that live less than a year to the human species, which has a maximum life span of more than a century. Even among primates maximum life spans vary by a factor of more than 10. The survival of most individual animals, however, does not approach the maximum species life spans.

There are several considerations that enter into animal survival (Hart and Turtarro, 1987). One is the minimum period required to achieve sexual maturity and reproduce. This is a requirement for species survival, but only a small percentage of individuals of high fecundity need survive to a reproductive age to assure the survival of the species. For short-lived species living under conditions that preclude reproduction during part of the year, some life cycle stage is required for species survival during the part of the year when reproduction cannot occur. For birds and mammals, reproductive success includes survival during a period required for the raising of young.

Three patterns of population survival, with variations, can be distinguished within the animal kingdom, as shown in Figure 1-1.

Survival curve A, which is concave in shape and describes a first-order reaction, applies to the survival in the wild of small animals that are low in the food chain, incapable of much useful adaptive and defensive behavior, and subject to high rates of exogenous killing from predation and environmental factors. Such curves have been published, for example, for the survival of small birds (Deevey, 1947) and rodents (Comfort, 1979), and a similar survival has been observed for untempered drinking glasses washed by machine in a restaurant (Comfort, 1979). In pattern A, the mortality of individuals is a largely random event, with its

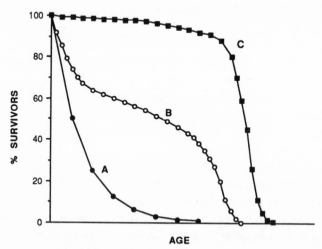

**Figure 1-1.** Three model survival curves. As discussed in the text, three curves, designated A, B, and C, describe three patterns of animal survival. The x-axis, which indicates age, is different for each animal species.

probability and rate remaining quite constant through the life span of a cohort. The death rate does not increase with age because the individuals do not reach an age that has an adverse effect on the ability to survive. It is doubtful that hominids ever had a survival curve like A.

Variations of curve B are seen in animals that, in adult life, have a period of reduced vulnerability to mortality. Curve B is complex, with two inflection points and with variable mortality rates. There is a large and largely random early die-off, represented by a curve such as A, but that does not involve the entire population. This is followed by a middle period with a lower death rate. Finally, there is an exponential increase in the death rate in later life. This exponentially increasing death rate with age in humans was first described early in the nineteenth century by the English actuary, Benjamin Gompertz. Populations described by curve B show *senescence*, which may be defined as a death rate that increases with age.

Among wild populations, physical changes, functional decrements, and sometimes even behavioral changes are recognized to explain the increased mortality in later life, as even marginally disadvantaged individuals are culled from the population. There are problems in constructing survival curves for naturally occurring populations. Early die-off cannot be assessed, and the time axis of survival curves begins well after birth or hatching. Curves of survival in the wild are based on three kinds of evidence: (a) postmortem remains on which age at death can be determined, (b) samples of survivors of an initial population taken at later times, for example, banded birds, and (c) the age structure, when age can be determined accurately, of a population observed at a fixed time.

Difficulties notwithstanding, type B curves have been observed in wild populations of several animal species, including the dall sheep and the herring gull (Deevey, 1947). As will be detailed, this type of curve described human survival of the past and still describes human survival in many countries. Some individuals in the animal studies of wild populations survive up to five times the mean life span for the population and must be regarded as reaching an advanced age.

Survival of a population can be altered from curves A and B in the direction of curve C by providing sheltered environments, such as are available to laboratory and zoo animals, and to domesticated animals that are not subject to harvest at young ages but are allowed to live as long as they can. Perinatal die-off, which may involve cannibalism, can be assessed with variable accuracy. Predation can be greatly reduced or eliminated, and environmental death through starvation, drought, freezing, and the like can be eliminated. Veterinary care can be provided, and even pathogen-free colonies have been established of some laboratory rodents.

Survival curve C has a convex shape. Most individuals survive to approximately the same advanced age, at which the death rate increases exponentially with age until the cohort has all died. These survival curves are sometimes described as rectangular or rectangularized. Most records of maximum life span are from such sheltered environments, and it is only in such environments that sufficient numbers survive to approach the maximum species life span.

Selected records of mammalian maximum life span are shown in Table 1-1, which is divided into credible records for wild animals in zoos, for domesticated animals that are commonly allowed to live through their natural life spans, and for laboratory animals that have been kept in sufficient numbers to the ends of their natural lives. The zoo records provide no information about the sexes of the animals, the conditions under which they were kept, or the causes of death. Zoo records are available for many more species than are shown in the Table, and the interested reader is referred to the admirable section on animal longevity in Comfort's (1979) *The Biology of Senescence* and to the other tabulations of maximum animal life spans (Altman and Dittmer, 1972; Committee on Animal Models for Research in Aging, 1981; Baker and Sprott, 1988; Finch, 1990) for additional values and discussion. Zoo life span records may cease to increase. In 1978, the American Association of Zoological Parks and Aquariums adopted a resolution to discourage the tendency toward unnatural prolongation of life of some animals in the effort to achieve "longevity records."

Some records far exceed the longevities of even the most longevous decile or percentile of a species kept under sheltered conditions, making them difficult to understand. An example is provided by the record of mouse (*Mus musculus*) survival (not indicated in Table 1-1) at the Jackson Laboratory, in Bar Harbor, Maine (Harrison and Archer, 1987). The most longevous mouse was of a long-lived genotype, being an $F_1$ hybrid (B6CBAFl) between C57BL/6J(B6) females and CBA/CaHT6J (CBA) males, and it was maintained under food restriction, which, as will be discussed (see Chapter 6), prolongs life in these mice compared with ad libitum feeding. (The mouse was fed ad libitum from day 1,541 to the end of its life.) The mouse lived 1,742 days, compared with a mean survival of 1,185 days in the experiment. Of 200 male mice in the experiment, the next longest lived individual lived 1,432 days, as is usually seen as a maximum life span of these mice. It is difficult to see the continuity of life span distribution in such a record, of an individual that exceeded the longevity of the most longevous percentile by 22 percent, which was nearly a year. As will be described later in this chapter, the current record of human longevity also shows a discontinuity with other data concerning the human maximum life span.

Such results raise a question about whether survival curve C, as shown in Figure 1-1, approaches the x-axis at an ever-accelerating rate, or whether large populations include a few individuals that do not share the senescence of most in the population. Their probability of dying seems to level off at the oldest ages

**Table 1-1. Records of Mammalian Longevity**

| Species | Years | Months |
|---|---|---|
| Zoo Animals | | |
| Marsupials | | |
| Northern oppossum | 4 | 10 |
| Tasmanian devil | 8 | 2 |
| Matschie's tree kangeroo | 15 | 7 |
| New South Wales koala | 17 | 0 |
| Rodents | | |
| Common field mouse | 4 | 5 |
| Plains pocket gopher | 7 | 2 |
| American beaver | 15 | 10 |
| Carnivores | | |
| Siberian weasel | 8 | 10 |
| Coyote | 21 | 10 |
| Bengal tiger | 26 | 3 |
| Polar bear | 34 | 7 |
| Bats | | |
| Pallid bat | 4 | 9 |
| Fisherman bat | 11 | 6 |
| Indian fruit bat | 31 | 5 |
| Ungulates (five mammalian oldels included) | | |
| Dorcas gazelle | 17 | 1 |
| Collard peccary | 24 | 7 |
| American bison | 26 | 0 |
| Scottish red deer | 26 | 8 |
| South American tapir | 35 | 0 |
| River hippopatamus | 54 | 4 |
| Asiatic elephant | 69 | 0 |
| Insectivores | | |
| European shrew | 0 | 3 |
| American mole | 1 | 11 |
| Short-nosed elephant shrew | 4 | 2 |
| Romanian hedgehog | 7 | 0 |
| Primates | | |
| Sportive lemur | 8 | 7 |
| Common squirrel monkey | 15 | 3 |
| Crab-eating macaque | 31 | 1 |
| White-faced capuchin monkey | 46 | 11 |
| Lowland gorilla | 47 | 11 |
| Chimpanzee | 53 | 0 |
| Laboratory Animals | | |
| Mice, DBA2/J | 2 | 10 |
| Mice, BALB/cAnNBd$_f$ | 3 | 2 |
| Rats, Fischer 344 (pathogen free) | 2 | 10 |
| Syrian hamsters | 2 | 2 |
| Guinea pigs | 6 | 8 |
| Domesticated Animals | | |
| Dogs, beagles | 19 | |
| Cats | <30 | |
| Horses | >40 | |

*Sources*: Altman and Dittmer, 1972; Comfort, 1979; Committee on Animal Models for Research in Aging, 1981; Baker and Sprott, 1988.

(Baringa 1991). This small number of outlyers probably constitutes some of the records of maximum species longevity.

Even casual perusal of animal longevity records reveals a relationship that has been confirmed by detailed analysis (e.g., Prothero and Jürgens, 1987). Larger animals live longer than smaller animals. This is seen within the mammalian orders, with kangaroos living longer than opossums, beavers living longer than mice, and tigers living longer than weasels. There are many exceptions to this generalization, with the value of the regression of size on record species life span being about 0.7 and with some animals exceeding the maximum life span predicted from their weights by a factor of two. An interesting exception is found within the species constituting the domesticated dog, of which there are many breeds that are capable of interbreeding. Smaller breeds, such as Pekinese and terriers, live longer than wolfhounds and mastifs (Comfort, 1960). Bats live longer than other mammals of comparable size, and marsupials live less long (Austad and Fischer, 1991). Birds live longer than mammals of comparable size, with some parrots and some birds of prey having record longevities of 40 to 50 years (Comfort, 1979; Finch, 1990).

Primates live longer than other mammals of comparable size, and a better correlation of a physical characteristic with maximum species life spans than total body mass is the proportion of the body mass that is brain[1] (*encephalization*) (Sacher, 1978). Humans are at the zenith of the relationship between maximum life span and encephalization.

There are also correlates of maximum species life span with characteristics of the life history (Promislow and Harvey, 1990). Species with longer life spans are less fecund, tend to mature later, give birth to larger offspring in fewer numbers after longer gestation, and have lower juvenile mortality than short-lived species. These differences are seen even after correction for size. In its life history characteristics, as in its encephalization and longevity, the human species is unique.

A conclusion commonly made from the diversity of maximum animal life spans, as shown in Table 1-1, is that maximum species life spans have genetic determinants. One can argue about whether the life spans in the table are records that will remain indefinitely, but there is no doubt that there are longer- and shorter-lived species, and maximum species life span is a characteristic that is transmitted from generation to generation (see Chapter 6).

Our coverage continues with an emphasis on human longevity, which is longer and different from that of any other mammal.

---

1. $\log L = 0.64 (\log E) - 0.23 (\log S) + 1.035$,
where $L$ = maximum life span; $E$ = adult brain weight; $S$ = adult body weight (Sacher, 1978).

## The Human Species: From Survival to Longevity

The current longevity of the U.S. population was described at the beginning of this chapter, and similar longevity patterns are shown for other economically developed countries. This was not always the case, and it is not the case today in most of the less-developed countries.

### Humans of the Past

Age determinations on skeletal remains of early humans reveal that some individuals lived into their 50s (Weidenreich, 1939; Vallois, 1961). In the case of the Chinese *Pithocanthropines*, it is possible that skull suture closure, the principal criterion for age determinations on skeletal material, occurred at a younger age than in modern humans and that age estimates are too great. Estimates of ages of Neanderthal, Paleolithic, and Mesolithic skeletal remains are more likely to be accurate, based on criteria for skeletal ages of modern humans. The majority of skeletons of early hominids (Simons, 1989) that have been found are of children and juveniles, and individuals estimated to have died in their 50s account for less than 5 percent of the remains. The skeletons indicate violent deaths from blows to the head and decapitation, and that cannibalism were common. Although the maximum life span experienced by early humans appears to have been less than half that of contemporary humans, it must be recognized that hominids were relatively long-lived animals as much as 100,000 years ago.

Individuals lived to greater ages in the Egyptian, Greek, and Roman civilizations. Based on papyrus writings, the Egyptians described the maximum human life span as 110 years, and specific individuals were described as living into their 80s (Zeman, 1942). It is likely that individuals lived at least into their 80s in classic Greece (Hansen, M.H., 1986), and Aristotle made some derogatory remarks about old men, although the age of his subjects is not known (Howell, 1988). Three percent of Roman funerary inscriptions in Italy describe persons more than 100 years of age, but ages appear to have been exaggerated (Hopkins, 1966). In the Roman colonies in North Africa a funerary inscription describes someone 82 years old (Durand, 1960), and skeletal remains of people of advanced ages were found in a Roman settlement in Romania (Fries, 1983).

It is impossible to interpret the Biblical descriptions of antediluvian patriarchs said to have lived more than 900 years, but individuals surely reached the threescore and ten years described in the Psalms. It is worth pondering the verse from Psalm 90 that describes the human life span as 70 years. The second half of the verse is less familiar than the first. "The days of our lives are threescore and ten; and if by reason of strength they be fourscore years, yet is their strength labor and sorrow, for it is soon cut off, and we fly away" (Psalm 90:10).

Excavations of Medieval cemeteries reveal skeletal remains from individuals in their 60s (Russell, 1987).

By the time of the Renaissance in Western Europe, reasonably systematic records, which are extant, were kept of births, marriages, and deaths, and there were even rudimentary attempts at census taking. It is possible to determine more about human life spans than is possible from earlier times when there are only records and skeletal remains to describe the age at death of isolated individuals. Historical demographers have used this information to estimate life expectancies of populations and to describe the age structures of populations, with some results shown in Table 1-2. Mean life expectancy at birth is estimated to have been around 30 years in the sixteenth, seventeenth, and eighteenth centuries (Vinovskis, 1971; Laslett, 1985, Knodel, 1988). The life expectancy at the age of 30, however, was another 30 or more years, and the young adult had a prospect of an adult life of considerable length, having survived the causes of death of infancy, childhood, and adolescence. It is estimated that a woman born in England in the seventeenth century had, at age 60, a mean life expectancy of another 12 years. Between 5 and 10% of several populations were over 60, but it

**Table 1-2.  Life Expectancy Estimates, Sixteenth, Seventeenth, and Eighteenth Centuries**

| Location and Year | Age | Life Expectancy at Age |
|---|---|---|
| England | | |
| 1541 | Birth | 33.7 |
| 1601 | Birth | 35.0 |
| 1661 | Birth | 35.9 |
| 1721 | Birth | 32.5 |
| 1781 | Birth | 34.7 |
| 1690s women | Birth | ca. 35 |
| | 30 | ca. 30 |
| | 50 | ca. 18 |
| | 60 | ca. 12 |
| | 70 | ca.  8 |
| Massachusetts (United States) | | |
| 1789 | Birth | 28 |
| | 5 | 41 |
| | 10 | 39 |
| | 30 | 30 |
| | 50 | 21 |
| | 60 | 15 |
| | 70 | 10 |
| | 80 | 6 |
| | 90 | 4 |

*Sources*: Vinovskis, 1971; Laslett, 1985.

is thought that figures describing 1 to 2% of populations as over 75 or 80 years reflect a tendency to exaggerate the ages of the very elderly (Laslett, 1985).

The specter of early death, sudden death, and short life still hung heavily over Renaissance society, reinforced by periodic plagues and epidemics and by the frequent death of young friends and family members. In 1517, at the age of 42, Michelangelo wrote to the business agent of his Medici patrons, "Besides I am old" (Gilbert, 1967). Perhaps this was a shrewd and useful posture for negotiation, but it must have been credible. He lived to be 89. Erasmus, who would live to be 70, wrote his poem "On the Discomforts of Old Age" at age 40. It is a lament that "dried up old age tires the body's strength" shortly after the "seventh five-year-span." Perhaps Dante Allegheri saw the matter more realistically when he wrote the *Divine Comedy* in his mid-30s and described "the middle of the road of our life." He would die at age 56.

Table 1-2 shows that life expectancy at birth changed little in Western Europe during the sixteenth, seventeenth, and eighteenth centuries. It increased considerably during the nineteenth century. Good records of sizeable populations, sometimes national populations, are available from that time, permitting the construction of life tables.

Increases in life expectancies at birth during the nineteenth century in several European national populations and in the state of Massachusetts are shown in Table 1-3. During that century, the life expectancy at birth increased from less than 40 years to about 50 years in several countries. This was an increase of more than a decade during the century. Factors contributing to the increase are discussed in the next chapter.

An interesting contrast to the life expectancy estimates from the United States and Western Europe is provided by a study of the demographics of the 3,500 serfs on the Pokrovskoe estate belonging to the Gagarin family in mid-nineteenth century Tsarist Russia. It is estimated that the mean life expectancy at birth was 25 years for women and 30 years for men (Hoch, 1986). It is estimated that 45 percent of those born were dead by age five.

## Life Span in the Twentieth Century

*Rapidly Developing Countries*

Comparison of the survival curves during the twentieth century, using the United States as an example, reveals three kinds of changes (Fig. 1-2). First, the mean life expectancy at birth has increased from about 50 years in 1900 to 75 years (average for both sexes) in 1989. Second, the shape of the survival curve has changed during the twentieth century from that described as type B to the rect-

Table 1-3.   Life Expectancies in the Nineteenth Century

| Country and Year | Life Expectancy at Birth (years) |
|---|---|
| England and Wales | |
| 1838–1854 | 40.9 |
| 1871–1880 | 43.0 |
| 1881–1890 | 45.4 |
| 1891–1900 | 46.0 |
| France | |
| 1817–1831 | 39.6 |
| 1840–1859 | 40.1 |
| 1861–1865 | 39.8 |
| 1877–1881 | 42.1 |
| 1898–1903 | 47.4 |
| Sweden | |
| 1816–1840 | 41.5 |
| 1841–1845 | 44.3 |
| 1846–1850 | 43.5 |
| 1851–1855 | 42.6 |
| 1856–1860 | 42.3 |
| 1861–1870 | 44.6 |
| 1871–1880 | 47.0 |
| 1881–1890 | 50.0 |
| 1891–1900 | 52.3 |
| Massachusetts (U.S.A.) | |
| 1855 | 39.8 |
| 1890 | 43.5 |
| 1895 | 45.3 |
| 1901 | 47.8 |

*Source*: Dublin, 1922.

angular curve described as type C. The die-off during the first year of life has fallen from about 15% of births to about 1%. Most people live long lives, and most deaths occur in individuals close to the mean life expectancy.

Third, two phases can be distinguished in the changing shape of twentieth century survival curves. The reduction of mortality in early life was largely complete as early as 1950. During the period from 1900 to 1950 the percentage of the population reaching the age of 20 increased from about 75 to 95.4%. It was approaching a limit, therefore, by 1980 it was 97.8% (Preston et al., 1972; National Center for Health Statistics, 1990). In 1900, only 4.6% of the population reached age 85. In 1950, it was calculated that 15.8% would reach 85, and this had doubled to 31% by 1980. The increased life survival since 1950 has involved mostly the prolongation of life of the elderly.

Table A-1 (Appendix) compares mean life expectancies at several ages in the populations of most of the economically developed countries. The data come

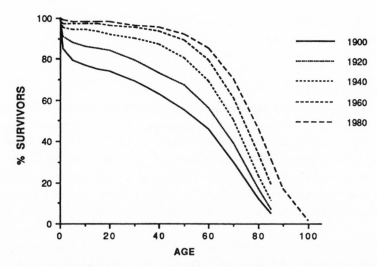

**Figure 1-2.** Survival curves in the United States since 1900. Based on life tables from the years shown, the percent survivors at each age are plotted. Referring to Figure 1-1, one can see the survival pattern changing from a curve B to a curve C type during the twentieth century. (Sources: Preston et al., 1972; National Center for Health Statistics, 1985, 1990.)

from the *Demographic Yearbook, 1988* (United Nations, 1990). There is some variation in the currency of the data, which are based on information reported by each country. The table includes only selected information, and much more complete information is available in the *Demographic Yearbook.*

The United States is about average among developed nations in life expectancy. In general, life expectancies are greater in wealthier European nations than in poorer ones, and life expectancies were shorter in Eastern Europe than in Western Europe in the 1980s. Women have greater life expectancies at every age than men in all economically developed countries (see Chapter 5). Neonatal and infant mortality are low, as indicated by greater life expectancies at birth than at one year of age, although there are a few exceptions, even in developed countries. Japan has the greatest life expectancies of all national populations for both men and women at every age. Japan surpassed Sweden in national longevity in the early 1980s (Svanborg et al., 1985), but the Japanese were not a long-lived population until after World War II. There were large increases during the 1950s, but in 1940, the mean life expectancy at birth (both sexes) was about 50 years in Japan compared with nearly 70 years in Sweden. Earlier in the twentieth century New Zealand was the longest lived nation (Dublin, 1922).

There is, of course, much heterogeneity within national populations, and there have been efforts to study the survival of smaller populations that are more homogeneous. Such studies, which are discussed in Chapter 4, give clues to the determinants of longevity.

*Less-Developed Nations*

Table A-2 shows life expectancies at several ages in countries that are in various stages of modernization and economic development and considered less developed than the countries listed in Table A-1. Again the data come from the *Demographic Yearbook, 1988* (United Nations, 1990), and were supplied by the countries themselves. It should be noted that the data are earlier, in general, than those from developed countries. Many countries evidently did not supply complete data, therefore, very limited information was available for inclusion in the table.

Life expectancies at birth in less-developed countries vary from less than 40 years to some values that are close to the life expectancies at birth in developed countries. In most of these countries, expectancies of remaining life are greater at several years of age than at birth—usually greater at five years, and often at 10 years. Although not shown in the table, mean life expectancy (years remaining) is greater at age 15 in Swaziland and at age 20 in Mali and Malawi than at birth. This pattern is reminiscent of life expectancies of the past in Western Europe and America. Indices of socioeconomic development, such as literacy and per capita income, seem to be better correlates of greater life expectancies in these less-developed countries than the level of public health (Rogers and Wofford, 1989).

Survival curves described as type B (see Fig. 1-1) are characteristic of less-developed countries, as they were of all human survival of the past. Figure 1-3 shows survival curves for the populations of two less-developed countries. The die-off in early life ranges up to 25 percent of those born.

On the other hand, those living to age 65 in some of these countries have mean life expectancies of 10 to 15 more years, which are not much less than the life expectancies of residents of developed countries at this age.

A few nations, such as Cuba and Sri Lanka, which are not usually considered as economically fully developed, have patterns of life expectancy at birth and at more advanced ages similar to those of developed countries.

*Records of Human Longevity*

As with the maximum species life spans of animals, one must look at rare cases—outlyers—for records of the maximum human life span.

The tendency noted previously to exaggerate the ages of the elderly may persist in our society. A critical consideration of claims of human longevity is provided by Comfort (1979). Documentation of the date of birth, date of death,

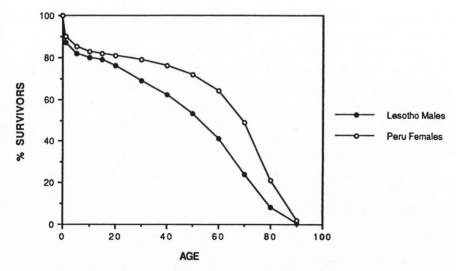

**Figure 1-3.** Recent survival curves in two less-developed countries. Based on life tables, the curves represent the survival of men in Lesotho in the mid-1970s and women in Peru in 1972. (Sources: Timaeus, 1984; Moses, 1985)

and continuity of identity all are necessary, and are usually not available. In *Vital Statistics of the United States, 1986* (National Center for Health Statistics, 1988) it is noted that one person died in 1986 at age 121, four at 120, one at 119, two at 118, and so on, for a total of 101 dying at age 110 and older. It appears that most of these records are not widely accepted for lack of documentation, although the ages were noted on the death certificates. Some even may represent careless errors in completing certificates (see Chapter 2).

A few years ago, records of longevity up to 130 years were alleged for residents of mountainous regions in the Caucuses, Tibet, and Ecuador, but eventually so much doubt was shed on these claims that they are no longer taken seriously (Leaf, 1990). Some of the individuals were quite old and in good physical condition, but it is doubtful that any was as old as claimed. Age had probably been exaggerated, and there may have been advantages to claiming advanced age to a military conscriptor or perhaps to a tax collector of the past—a claim that the claimant sometimes had to live with for the rest of his life.

The record for well-documented human longevity is held by Shigichio Izumi, a Japanese man who died on Kyushu in 1986 at the age of 120 (*Guinness Book of World Records*, 1987). He was recorded as one-year-old in the Japanese census of 1867, and acceptance of his stated age was evidenced by his designation as a "Living National Treasure" by the Japanese government. As with the record of mouse longevity noted previously, this record of human longevity was established by an outlyer, and it is difficult to consider it on a continuum of human longevity. The record is two decades beyond the century mark, which was reached by few people in the past. It is estimated that 1.5 percent of those born today will reach the century mark. There are a few other reasonably well-authenticated records of human longevity between 110 and 115 years (Comfort, 1979). There is an accepted record of a Canadian woman who died in 1986 at 114 (Metropolitan Life, 1987a), and in 1990, newspaper accounts appeared of the death of an American man at age 112 who is said to have had a birth certificate.

It can be argued that there is no way the criterion of identity continuity could be fully satisfied by the very old of today. Fingerprints or footprints appear on some more modern birth certificates and will allow the authentication of identity in the future. A molecular marker may someday be used to establish the identity of long-lived individuals with certainty.

## Conclusions and Questions

This chapter has described human life spans as they were in the past and as they are today, when the mean life expectancy at birth in the United States is about 72 years for men and 79 years for women. Many people live well beyond these ages, but the maximum life span for the human species is approached only rarely. Mean life expectancy at birth has approximately doubled during the past two centuries and has increased approximately 50 percent since 1900. Similar changes have occurred in the other economically developed countries.

Several questions occur in considering human longevity, and the logical organization of the remainder of this volume is the exploration of these questions.

What caused these changes in the human life span? The changes have much to do with changing causes of death. With economic development we have changed from a species with many individuals dying at young ages to one with most individuals dying at advanced ages of different causes. Causes of death of the very old are sometimes obscure and may not be recognizable as the common causes of mortality of younger elderly people. Is there such a thing as mortality associated with old age without underlying fatal disease (see Chapter 2)?

What are the biomedical factors limiting the life spans of humans? These factors may operate through the development of fatal disease, but factors causing mortality without fatal disease at advanced ages must also be considered. Comparison of the maxiumum life span of the human species with maximum life spans of other animal species leads to the conclusion that life spans are genetically determined. What are the genes that act to determine life spans of humans and other animals (see Chapter 3)?

Societal and behavioral factors act to determine life span by reducing the amount of the potential life span that is realized. The operation of these factors shows great variation in different human populations. What are some of these factors (see Chapter 4)?

A phenomenon recognizable in this chapter is that, on the average, women live longer than men. Why? Some explanations are soundly based on mammalian sexual development and the pathogenesis of diseases that are major causes of death. Some are based on realities of human societies. Some are attractive additional explanations that must be regarded as speculative at present (see Chapter 5).

From an evolutionary point of view, the human species occupies a unique position as the most longevous of all warm-blooded animals. We are a species with a requirement for long life just for species survival, but our maximum species life span exceeds the minimum for species survival by a factor of three or four. Why can humans live so long? What about evolution and life span determination in shorter lived mammals? How might the evolution of a long human life span have been favored by natural selection (see Chapter 6)?

What is happening to human longevity? Human life expectancy continues to increase, and there are sound reasons to expect this increase to continue for many more years. A consequence is that ever more people will reach advanced ages. The maximum human life span as it is established today will be tested as it is approached by greater numbers of individuals. There will be more outlyers as 1.5 percent of those born live to 100 years and beyond. Is there any possibility that the maximum human life span will be extended, not marginally by increased numbers of outlyers, but by the operation of new limiting factors (see Chapter 7)?

A brief final chapter summarizes the answers to these questions as they can be considered today.

# 2

# Causes of Death

Perhaps in the case of certain maladies a diseased state of the body and shortness of life are interchangeable, while in cases of others, ill-health is perfectly compatible with long life.

ARISTOTLE, 384–322 B.C.
On the Length and Shortness of Life

As described previously, the mean human life expectancy in the United States has increased about 50 percent during this century. Contemporary Americans and residents of other developed countries no longer survive, but commonly live to ages approaching the maximum human life span and experience what can be called both longevity and senescence (see Chapter 1). What has happened, and how has it happened? The answers have something to do with changing causes of human death. Life continues until the individual encounters some fatal event, and our abilities to avoid fatal events and to survive potentially fatal events individually and as a population have changed.

## Causes of Death in the United States in 1900

A comparison of the major causes of death in contemporary United States with those at the beginning of the century is instructive. Although that time seems remote to most of us, it is within the memory of some persons still living, and there are reasonably good records of what the United States was like at that time. Table 2-1 lists the major causes of death and their rates per 100,000 Americans as reported in 1900 (Bureau of Foreign and Domestic Commerce, 1914). The annual mortality rate in 1900 was 1,755 persons per 100,000, which is twice the 1986 rate of 873 per 100,000. The system of classifying causes of death in 1900 was very different from that of today, and as discussed later, commonly indicated the organ or system in which the disease was manifested. It is uncertain what constituted an acceptable entry on the death certificate, and undoubtedly many died unattended by a physician.

**Table 2-1.  Principal Causes of Death, 1900**

| Cause | Deaths per 100,000 |
|---|---|
| Respiratory diseases (not including pulmonary tuberculosis and influenza) | 256 |
| Digestive diseases | 224 |
| Central nervous system diseases | 204 |
| Pulmonary tuberculosis | 182 |
| Circulatory diseases | 147 |
| Genitourinary diseases | 106 |
| Accidents | 79 |
| Malignant tumors | 64 |
| Diphtheria and croup | 43 |
| Typhoid and paratyphoid | 36 |
| Influenza | 23 |
| Other tuberculosis | 20 |
| Other infectious diseases | 19 |
| Measles | 12 |
| Whooping cough | 12 |
| Suicide | 11 |
| Scarlet fever | 10 |
| Diabetes mellitus | 10 |
| Not listed above | 284 |
| Death rate in 1900 | 1,755 |

*Source*: Bureau of Foreign and Domestic Commerce, 1914.

A little additional information not in Table 2-1 can be reconstructed from other sources. Most significantly, it is estimated that in 1900 there were 3,230 live births per 100,000 people, and that 16 percent of infants died within the first year of life (Bureau of the Census, 1975), accounting for 500 deaths per 100,000—nearly one-third of all deaths. Figures from 1915, when such information was recorded (Bureau of the Census, 1975), indicate that nearly half of these infant deaths occurred in the neonatal period, which is defined as the first seven days of life. It is uncertain how much of the neonatal and infant mortality was tabulated as respiratory and digestive diseases. The maternal mortality rate in 1900 was estimated to be 6.1 per 1,000 births (Bureau of the Census, 1975), which means that the maternal death rate per 100,000 persons was 19.1, a more significant cause of death than some listed in Table 2-1. The reader's attention is called to the 284 deaths per 100,000 from causes not on the list.

The data in Table 2-1 come from death certificates from states in which such records were required. In 1900, the so-called registration states were Maine, Vermont, New Hampshire, Massachusetts, Rhode Island, Connecticut, New York, New Jersey, Delaware, the District of Columbia, Michigan, and Indiana. These states, all in the Northeast, represented the most urbanized part of the

United States, and included only about 40 percent of the total U.S. population in 1900. No Southern states were included, and vital statistics were reported on few black Americans. It was not until 1933 that all states were required to register births and deaths. The decennial census data from 1900 do not even provide death rates for nonregistration states.

The practice of medicine has changed greatly since 1900, and without getting into a detailed consideration of medical history, it is worth consulting Osler's *Principles and Practice of Medicine*, fourth edition (Osler, 1901), to find out what the listed causes of death meant at that time. This book represented the state of the art in diagnosing and interpreting the items listed as the principal causes of death, and its contents probably far exceeded the understanding and expertise of most individuals completing death certificates in 1900. Although it is fair to say that in 1900 the medical profession could not do much in the face of most diseases, there were some intellectual strengths. These were based on the autopsies performed in the second half of the nineteenth century, which gave a clear picture of the pathology underlying many clinical presentations, and the bacteriology of the same period in which many bacterial pathogens were identified, isolated, and characterized.

Of the entities listed in Table 2-1, pulmonary tuberculosis was the most common single cause of death. As a disease it was well understood in 1900, and awareness and agreement were at a high level. Osler (1901) stated, "Tuberculosis is the most universal scourge of the human race." The item listed as "Other tuberculosis" included more obscure conditions such as tuberculous meningitis and tuberculous abscesses of visceral organs, and many cases were probably missed. "Respiratory diseases not including pulmonary tuberculosis and influenza" included a variety of disorders that had failure and usually inflammation of the respiratory system as a common feature. It included a variety of pneumonias of infants and children, and it also included the lobar pneumonia of elderly people, usually caused by the *Pneumococcus* bacteria. Osler (1901) described the annual death rate from lobar pneumonia as 734 per 100,000 persons over the age of 65. He wrote, "Pneumonia may well be called the friend of the aged. Taken off by it in an acute, short, not often painful illness, the old man escapes those 'cold gradations of decay' so distressing to himself and to his friends."

Digestive diseases, another of the major causes of death, include a variety of conditions that have in common malfunction and usually inflammation of the digestive system. Much infant and childhood mortality is included in this category, and infant and childhood diarrhea remains a major cause of death today in many less-developed countries (discussed later). In 1900, diarrhea led to dehydration, which could not be treated at that time, and was fatal.

Table 2-1 includes the following additional infectious diseases: syphilis, typhoid and paratyphoid, scarlet fever and strep throat, diphtheria, whooping cough, and measles. Accidents and suicide were also major causes of death.

Circulatory diseases were a major cause of death in 1900. The category includes a variety of entities, and grouping them together is a serious oversimplification of the understanding of heart disease that existed in 1900. It is commonly stated that the myocardial infarct (heart attack) was first described in 1912 by Herrick (1912), and this paper probably clarified the correlation of clinical presentation with pathology. It is clear, however, both from the discussion in Herrick's paper (1912) and from Osler (1901), that most of the pieces of the puzzle were understood well before 1912. These included angina pectoris (chest pain referable to the heart and now known to be associated with oxygen deficiency of the myocardium), which was known to terminate fatally sometimes. Sclerosis of the coronary arteries was well known, and diabetes mellitus was recognized as a risk factor. Experimental studies had been done on occlusion of the coronary arteries in laboratory animals. Heart failure was understood, and rheumatic heart disease, bacterial endocarditis, and various congenital malformations of the heart had been well described.

Among diseases of the central nervous system, strokes and apoplexy resulting from thrombosis and emboli in the arteries of the brain were well understood. In considering kidney diseases, acute and chronic nephritis were well understood, including associations with streptococcal infections and with hypertension.

The major malignant tumors had been described. The low incidence of cancer shown in the Table 2-1 reflects both the relative scarcity of elderly people in 1900 and the fact that 1900 predated most of the procedures now available for the diagnosis of cancer. Many cases were probably confused with other things.

## Death Certificates

It is necessary that this chapter, as with any other discussion of causes of death, rely on information from death certificates, even though this information is badly flawed. Uncertainties resulting from the death certificates of the past continue in considering death certificates that are being completed today.

The idea of the death certificate was first introduced by the U. S. government in 1850, but in 1880 only Massachusetts, New Jersey, and the District of Columbia required them. In 1900, the registration states were as listed and still represented less than half of the population. Today's certification is administered at the level of the state government, and although the federal government recommends information that should be gathered and a form for doing so, the certificate forms vary from state to state (National Center for Health Statistics, 1988).

Some basic information is requested about the decedent, including sometimes marital status and usual occupation (before retirement). The physician completing the certificate (the certifier) is asked the relationship to the case. The certifier specifies the immediate cause of death and is asked for three or four conditions underlying the immediate cause of death and contributing to it. A sequence can be described, including the duration of each condition. Entries are according to the *International Classification of Diseases*, 9th edition (World Health Organization, 1977). The information from certificates is ultimately transmitted to the National Center for Health Statistics for tabulation according to a program for determining the underlying cause of death.

The information on death certificates provides a potential for the analysis of multiple cause of death data (Israel et al., 1986), but in tabulations a single underlying cause of death is assigned. Most entries in the *International Classification of Diseases* are very specific and reflect modern standards of diagnosis. As will be discussed later, however, the entities reflect limitations and are not always adequate to describe causes of death.

The tabulation of causes of death is dependent on the use of *The International Classification of Diseases*. One tabulation based on 72 selected causes of death leaves many cases that must be listed as "other causes of death" (National Center of Health Statistics, 1988), whereas another tabulation with 282 selected causes of death provides causes for all deaths. A residual category of "other causes of death" is not needed. Even more detailed is a tabulation based on all of the three-digit and some of the four-digit entities in the international classification. Although no broad residual category of "other causes" or "other diseases" results, there are residual categories of categories such as "other pericardial disease."

There is a category for the expression of uncertainty as to cause of death entitled "symptoms and signs, ill-defined." It is used for mortality that cannot be attributed to any underlying disease. Features, such as physical findings, symptoms, organ failure, and abnormal laboratory results, may be recorded on the death certificate. This category is not used very much, but it is used most often on the death certificates of the very young and the very old. Difficulty in establishing the cause of death in some very elderly people is discussed.

The quality of the data on death certificates obviously varies depending on the competence and the familiarity with the case of the certifier. Certificates in other developed countries seem to request similar information, but, as will be detailed, there appear to be national differences in the use of entities for classification. The use of residual categories appears to be more popular in some other developed countries than in the United States, as indicated by differences in recorded causes of death in national populations that would seem to be much alike (discussed later). It is even more difficult to interpret mortality data (described later) from less-developed countries where standards of medical practice are lower and where many people probably die without medical attention.

It must be recognized that death certificates have many purposes, only one of which is the provision of vital statistical information. They are also required for the release and disposition of bodies and as legal proof of death for probate and for claims on insurance and other assets. Death certificates are completed in haste, and stories exist of death certificates completed by funeral directors. A well-known medical examiner told the author that public policy should not be based on death certificate data because of its quality. Some entries may be questioned by state vital statistics agencies, but most are not. The autopsy rate in the United States is 12.6 percent of deaths (National Center for Health Statistics, 1988), but even when an autopsy has been done, the death certificate is not modified to reflect the autopsy findings. A sizeable literature indicates that 25 to 50 percent of causes of death recorded on death certificates are at serious variance with autopsy findings (e.g., James et al., 1955; Cameron and McGoogan, 1981; Kircher et al., 1985).

Thus, although data based on death certificates will appear frequently in this volume, this discussion constitutes a warning about the validity of such data.

## Causes of Death in Contemporary United States

Table 2-2 shows the principal causes of death in the United States in 1986. This table should be compared with Table 2-1, as the comparison emphasizes the

**Table 2-2. Principal Causes of Death, 1986**

| Cause | Deaths (per 100,000, not age-adjusted) |
|---|---|
| Major cardiovascular disease | 402 |
| Heart disease | 318 |
| Ischemic heart disease | 216 |
| Cerebrovascular disease | 62 |
| All malignant disease | 195 |
| Of the respiratory system | 54 |
| Of the gastrointestinal system | 48 |
| Of the genital organs | 21 |
| Of the breast | 17 |
| Leukemia | 7 |
| All accidents | 39 |
| Motor vehicle accidents | 20 |
| Chronic obstructive pulmonary disease | 32 |
| Pneumonia | 28 |
| Diabetes mellitus | 15 |
| Suicide | 13 |
| Chronic liver disease and cirrhosis | 11 |
| Not listed above | 138 |
| Total rate | 873 |

differences in the medical practice in 1900 and in the contemporary United States. The words to describe the principal causes of death have different meanings with, for example, the circulatory diseases of 1900 not being at all comparable to the cardiovascular diseases of 1986.

The death rate in 1986, 873 per 100,000 people, was half the rate in 1900. The mortality rate is much influenced today by the age structure of the population, and the death rate is now very low in younger age groups. The rates in the table are not age adjusted because the intent is to provide a comparison with 1900 as well as with other countries, and to describe rates as they were at the times shown rather than after adjustment to 1940 (see Chapter 1).

The rates shown in Table 2-2 are for the entire U.S. population, although, as discussed in Chapter 4, age-adjusted mortality rates for some of the major causes of death differ by factors of two or more in different states.

The list in Table 2-2 includes only broad categories and the major causes of death. Vastly more detail is available in *Vital Statistics of the United States, 1986* (National Center for Health Statistics, 1988).

The three major causes of death in the United States today are, in descending order, ischemic heart disease, cancer, and cerebrovascular disease (strokes). These diseases affect chiefly older people, and death rates from them increase strikingly with age, as shown in Figure 2-1. Along with other diseases, they

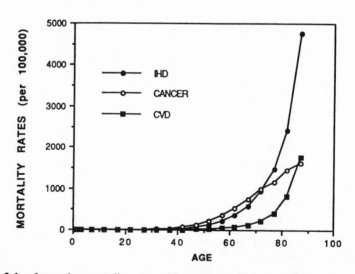

**Figure 2-1.** Increasing mortality rates with age for the three most common causes of death. Mortality rates at various ages are plotted for ischemic heart disease (IHD), cancer, and cerebrovascular disease (CVD), based on the United States population, 1986. (Source: National Center for Health Statistics, 1988.)

affected the elderly people of the past, but although persons 65 years and over account for about 12.5% of the population today, they accounted for only 4.0% of the population in 1900. In 1900, only about 40% of the population reached the age of 65 compared with 75% today (National Center for Health Statistics, 1988). Of deaths in 1986, only about 30% were of people under 65. Most people today are spared or survive the causes that used to kill people at younger ages and go on to die of the diseases of old age.

The specific infectious diseases listed in 1900 (Table 2-1) have all disappeared from the list of major causes of death in 1986. Of more than 2 million deaths in 1986, the total numbers of deaths from the former killer infectious diseases were as follows: diphtheria, 0 (one death from diphtheria was recorded in 1982); measles (rubeola), 2; measles (rubella) 1; whooping cough, 6; salmonellosis (compare with paratyphoid), 102; typhoid, 2; syphilis, 80; and tuberculosis (all forms) 1,782 (Centers for Disease Control, 1989a). Pneumonia is still on the list and remains a mixture of diseases. Gastroenteritis is no longer on the list.

Clinical tuberculosis is once again increasing, affecting primarily those with acquired immunodeficiency as an opportunistic infection and the poor in urban populations (Bloom and Murray, 1992). The increased incidence of clinical tuberculosis is not reflected on death certificates, and, in cases in which it is an opportunistic infection, it will not be listed as the cause of death.

Acquired immunodeficiency syndrome (AIDS), the new killer among infectious diseases (human immunodeficiency virus), was listed as the cause of 10,900 deaths in 1986 (Centers for Disease Control, 1989b). It is, therefore, not listed as a major cause of death in Table 2-2. It was a major cause of death for large groups within the population such as young men and women of child-bearing age (Chu et al., 1990). It was probably underreported because of complications such as opportunistic infections. Deaths from this cause had increased to 24,264 in 1989, which was nearly equal to the number of deaths attributed to chronic liver disease. Projections indicate that it may account for 53,000 to 75,000 deaths in 1993 (Centers for Disease Control, 1990).

## What Happened to Change the Causes of Death?

Part of the answer to this question lies in preventive medicine and medical practice. The microbiology of the second half of the nineteenth century and the early years of the twentieth century resulted in vaccines, antitoxins, and antisera to bacterial and viral pathogens. Measures were taken to reduce contagion. Milk was pasteurized and dairy herds were tuberculin tested. Later came the antibiotic era, when bacteriostatic and bactericidal drugs were produced that can usually save the patient, even in advanced cases of most bacterial diseases, and effective interventions were developed to save patients and prolong life in the face of other diseases.

The improvement of living standards in a broad sense has been even more important in increasing life expectancy (McKinlay and McKinlay, 1977), and, as discussed previously (see Chapter 1), the increase began in the nineteenth century, before there had been much advance in preventive medicine and medical practice. Much of the Western world prospered. People ate better, and the food supply was more certain. Most of the population received at least the rudiments of an education, and with education came awareness and healthier life styles. Personal and public hygiene improved.

In the United States during the period from 1860 to 1900, although medical practice changed little, as indicated by a quite constant level of infant mortality at 12 to 16% of live births, the death rate from pulmonary tuberculosis declined nearly 50%. Death rates from diphtheria and typhoid/paratyphoid declined by factors of 2 to 5, depending on which years are compared. Sporadic outbreaks of these diseases increased death rates transiently up through the early years of this century. The death rate from smallpox fell from a level of 3 to 20 per 100,000 (depending on the year) to 0.1 per 100,000. A vaccine for this disease had been available since approximately 1800, therefore, most of the decline in the smallpox death rate had actually occurred in the first half of the nineteenth century. Interestingly, the pathogenesis and viral etiology of smallpox were not understood at all in 1900, although an effective vaccine had been available for a century. The disease now appears to have disappeared worldwide.

## A Primer in Ischemic Heart Disease, Cancer, and Strokes

The section that follows is a brief presentation of essential information about ischemic heart disease, cancer, and strokes. The information is common knowledge to those who are medically trained, and it can be found in greater detail in any good textbook of medicine or pathology (e.g., Cotran et al., 1989; Wilson et al., 1991). It is intended for readers who are not medically trained as an aid in considering life span in the context of causes of death. The information is necessary for an understanding of not only this chapter but also subsequent chapters. These diseases have pathobiology that is largely unique to the human species, as will be discussed.

### Ischemic Heart Disease

The word *ischemia* means the relative lack of blood flow and implies circulatory insufficiency and the deficiency of oxygen. Of the nutrients delivered in the blood, a deficiency of oxygen is the first to result in cell malfunction and cell death. Ischemia may affect any organ, and the usual cause is arterial obstruction. This may be chronic, with gradual impingement on the arterial lumen by the lesions of atherosclerosis (discussed later), or it may be acute, with sudden occlusion of the arterial lumen by thrombosis (blood clotting). In the case of the heart, thrombosis usually occurs in coronary arteries already affected by atherosclerosis. Although not all ischemic heart disease is based on coronary artery disease, most of it is. The mortality rate from ischemic heart disease increases exponentially with age (see Fig. 2-1).

Even in the absence of atherosclerosis, larger arteries show gradual changes with age, including increased thickness of the intima (the innermost layer of the arterial wall), accumulation of smooth muscle cells and cholesterol in the intima, and increased rigidity of the vessel walls and perivascular tissues. Age-related changes in collagen, which will be discussed in the next chapter, contribute to the rigidity. The changes can be regarded as degenerative in that they are progressive with time and are not reversible, and they have been attributed to wear and tear. In atherosclerosis these changes are focally exaggerated with plaque-like lesions in the intima of large arteries. The plaques consist of accumulations of smooth muscle cells that become engorged with cholesterol. The process begins in adolescence in some individuals, and its occurrence and progression is highly variable. The plaques begin as fatty streaks consisting of a few lipid-engorged cells and enlarge and become more complex. There may be hemorrhage and calcification in the plaques that become largely acellular cholesterol accumulations, and plaque surfaces may ulcerate. The plaques impinge progressively on arterial lumens, and by the time the lumen of a coronary artery is 70 percent obstructed, symptoms of chronic coronary insufficiency and myocardial ischemia may appear, as manifested by angina pectoris, which is most likely to occur during exertion. Symptoms of angina pectoris include chest pain, discomfort, and shortness of breath. Although progression is usual in atherosclerotic disease, regression with increased coronary blood flow has been described (e.g., Brown et al., 1990).

Plaques predispose to thrombosis, and when this occurs in a major branch of the coronary circulation, the heart muscle supplied by this branch becomes acutely hypoxic and dies, resulting in a myocardial infarct. If enough of the myocardium dies, the heart will fail acutely as a pump, killing the individual. Alternatively, the electrical impulses necessary to pace and coordinate the pumping action of the heart may be disrupted by the necrotic muscle, or the necrotic and injured myocardium may set up aberrant ectopic foci of electrical activity, which may arrest the effective pumping action of the heart.

Heart muscle cells do not regenerate, and if an individual survives the acute myocardial infarct, the necrotic muscle undergoes liquifaction in the early stages of repair, with consequent weakening of the wall of the heart, which may rupture. The dead muscle is replaced by a scar consisting of fibroblasts and their extracellular product, collagen. The scar may restore a measure of structural integrity to the healing heart, but it is not muscle, and it does not contribute to the function of the heart as a pump. The remaining muscle cells may hypertrophy (increase in size) to compensate for the cell loss, but the injured heart may be compromised as a pump for the rest of the life of the individual.

Several risk factors have been identified in the development of ischemic heart disease and its complication of myocardial infarction. Calling them risk factors perhaps begs the questions of their actual causative roles and their mechanisms of causation, but most of the evidence for the risk factors is epidemiological (e.g., Castelli, 1984). Those that are most widely accepted are age (see Fig. 2-1), hyperlipidemia (high plasma lipids, discussed later), male sex (see Chapter 5), smoking, hypertension, and diabetes mellitus. Less well established as risk factors are overweight, physical inactivity, stress, and personality. Some of these risk factors result from life styles, which can be altered. Others are intrinsic, with some having genetic components that are discussed in Chapter 3.

The subject of hyperlipidemia is discussed repeatedly in this volume, therefore, it is worth considering hyperlipidemia briefly at this point. The public is well aware of the correlation of plasma cholesterol levels and heart attacks. There is also a correlation between high levels of plasma triglycerides (fats) and ischemic heart disease. The usual American diet contains about 100 g of fat (triglycerides) and about 1 g of cholesterol per day. These are absorbed in an emulsified form from the intestine and transported as small droplets, first in the lymphatic circulation and then in the blood, to muscle and fatty depots for energy and storage. Cholesterol is carried to the liver, which also synthesizes cholesterol endogenously from small precursor molecules derived from carbohydrate and protein metabolism, as well as from fats. In humans and in some animals there is a reciprocal relationship between cholesterol synthesis and cholesterol absorbed from the intestine, with the approximate level of plasma cholesterol being determined genetically (Vesselinovitch, 1988). Cholesterol, its deleterious effects not withstanding, is far from an unmitigated curse on mankind. Cholesterol and esterified cholesterol comprise the bile acids secreted by the liver, concentrated by the gallbladder, and expelled into the intestine, where they have a role in the emulsification and absorption of fat, other lipids, and the oil-soluble vitamins from the intestine. Almost all (95 percent) of the biliary cholesterol and cholesterol esters are resorbed and recycled to the liver. Thus, there are three sources of the cholesterol in the plasma: dietary cholesterol, endogenously synthesized cholesterol, and recycled (conserved) cholesterol. In addition to bile acids, cholesterol provides the basic chemical moiety of sex and adrenal steroid hormones, and it is incorporated into cell membranes. The plasma cholesterol level rises through childhood and young adult life, and in the population there is an approximately Gaussian distribution of plasma cholesterol values, with those below 200 mg/100 mL being regarded as low (< 5th percentile) and those over 270 mg/100 mL as high (> 95th percentile).

Plasma cholesterol is mostly in combination with specific proteins, which are called lipoproteins when carrying lipids. The two important forms of plasma cholesterol-carrying lipoproteins are called low-density lipoproteins (LDLs) and high-density lipoproteins (HDLs), based on their buoyant densities and on the nature of the associated protein molecules (apoproteins). Apoproteins of type A are in HDLs and apoproteins of type B are in LDLs. There is some heterogeneity in both the LDLs and HDLs. The level of LDLs correlates with the incidence of ischemic heart disease, and it is in this form that cholesterol enters arterial walls and is delivered to specific sites where it is used, such as the adrenal glands. Low-density lipoproteins are formed in the liver. High-density lipoproteins are formed in the peripheral tissues and represent cholesterol that is unused in those tissues and that is in transit back to the liver. There is a negative correlation between HDL levels and ischemic heart disease, and individuals with high levels may regard themselves as fortunate.

Patterns of plasma lipoproteins as well as levels of cholesterol and cholesterol synthesis are determined genetically (see Chapter 3), with some hormonal modification (see Chapter 5). A few monogenic conditions are recognized in which there is hypercholesterolemia and associated accelerated atherosclerosis and early death from myocardial infarction (see Chapter 3). Modification of levels is possible by diet and other life style factors, by drugs that prevent the resorption of the bile acids, and by drugs that reduce cholesterol synthesis in the liver (see Chapter 7). The cases of regression of atherosclerotic lesions have followed reductions in serum cholesterol.

## Cancer

Cancer is a disease of great heterogeneity. There are not only malignant tumors of every organ but also malignant tumors that are related to almost every kind of cell of which each organ is composed. The presentations and clinical courses of cancer as a disease are diverse. The incidence of many but not all diagnostic entities that can be called cancer increases with age, as does the death rate from cancer, as shown in Figure 2-1. In contrast to death rates from ischemic heart disease and cerebrovascular disease, which increase exponentially with age, the age-related increase of cancer deaths (all kinds of cancer) is approximately linear, as shown in the figure.

Cancer has as its common feature the progressive and uncontrolled proliferation of the cells involved, resulting in local spread, invasion, and often tumor growth in remote sites (metastasis). Environmental factors (e.g., carcinogenic chemicals and ionizing radiation), genetic factors as discussed in Chapter 3, and viruses have been implicated in some human neoplasms (cancer), but most cancer arising in humans is presently of obscure etiology. The strong association between smoking and bronchogenic cancer is not paralleled in most other forms of cancer. Cancer death may result from invasion of vital structures by the tumor, obstruction, wasting, and terminal infection.

Some kinds of malignant tumors are characteristic of younger individuals because it is only in these younger individuals that the cells of origin are present or that the hormonal environment is supportive of tumor cell proliferation. Thus, Wilms tumors (a tumor of embryonic kidney cells) are seen only in young children. Carcinoma of the esophagus and malignant melanoma of the skin have their peak incidence in younger adults. Death rates from cancers of the bowel and breast increase linearly with age, whereas carcinoma of the prostate has a striking predilection for old men, with the incidence of and death rate from this tumor increasing exponentially.

Why do the incidence and death rate from most cancers increase with age? There is evidence that most types of cancers arise from a single cell, and it is commonly accepted, based on experimental studies, that the process of carcino-genesis has multiple stages, with two or more events being involved in the initiation and promotion of the tumor. The probability that a cell may undergo all of the required steps increases with age. A clone of neoplastic cells has a tenuous existence in the body, with immune mechanisms able to destroy the cancer at an early stage. Gradual diminution in the function of the immune system with age, particularly near the end of the life span, is well documented (see Chapter 3), and thus endogenous defenses against the growth of cancer cells are decreased with age. It is estimated that the process of carcinogenesis from smoking requires 20 to 40 years. When smoking begins in the teens and twenties, the process com-monly runs its course before old age is reached. It is often the first experience with cancer that kills.

## Cerebrovascular Disease (Strokes)

Strokes are the consequences of thrombosis and embolization in the vasculature of the brain and of hemorrhages from these vessels. In 1901, Osler wrote, "thus the natural tendency to degeneration of the blood vessels in advanced life makes apoplexy much more common after the fiftieth year." Osler's observation of the age relatedness of strokes is well supported in data from the National Center for Health Statistics, as illustrated in Figure 2-1. Osler's comment on age and blood vessels was insightful. Death from strokes increases exponentially with age.

The brain is particularly vulnerable to ischemia, with only a momentary inter-ruption of arterial oxygen resulting in unconsciousness and only about three minutes resulting in irreversible brain death. Moreover, the softness of brain tissues offers little resistance to damage resulting from hemorrhage.

Atherosclerosis and the more generalized process called lipohyalinization occur in the cerebral arteries and their primary branches, and thrombosis is more likely to occur in the atherosclerotic vessels as a result of their narrowed lumens and a predisposition to clotting in the region of plaques. Emboli may form in the left side of the heart and in the more proximal vessels leading to the brain based on several mechanisms, including the formation of small thrombi on atheromatous plaques. If the thrombi become detached, they may be carried in the cerebral circulation until they reach a sufficiently small vessel to obstruct it. Cerebral hemorrhages occur because of hypertension and defects in vessel walls.

The clinical picture depends on the location of the lesion in the brain. Infarction or hemorrhage in parts of the brain that provide major functions or that carry major fiber tracts cause profound symptoms that may be incompatible with life or that may cause major disability. On the other hand, there are parts of the brain in which relatively extensive lesions are quite silent.

As with the heart, regeneration does not occur in the central nervous system. Neurons (nerve cells), once destroyed, are not replaced. Fiber tracts passing through necrotic areas are permanently disrupted. There is considerable redundancy in some functions of the central nervous system, therefore, some retraining may be possible. However, although strokes rank third as a cause of death in the United States, they rank first as a cause of disability.

The same risk factors and conditions that predispose to ischemic heart disease also predispose to cerebrovascular disease. Atherosclerosis is important in the pathogenesis of each, and hyperlipidemia, diabetes, smoking, age, and sex are risk factors in atherosclerosis. Hypertension is a factor in atherosclerosis and also in cerebral hemorrhages. It may be associated with other diseases, or it may be without associated disease (primary or essential hypertension). Risk factors include advanced age, black race, male sex, smoking, high cholesterol level, overweight, and diabetes. It has long been assumed to have a genetic component that is multifactorial, based both on animal studies (there are hypertensive mouse strains) and on familial correlations. Many cases of hypertension are aggravated by the consumption of salt (NaCl and perhaps calcium).

## Causes of Death in Other Countries

### Developed Countries

The *Demographic Yearbook, 1986* (United Nations, 1988) provides data on the principal causes of death in most developed countries, based on death certificates. The causes are classified according to the *International Classification of*

*Diseases*, with some countries using the eighth revision (World Health Organization, 1967) and some using the ninth revision (World Health Organization,
1977). Some inconsistencies are introduced by the use of two different classification systems, although each is based on the etiology of diseases.

Data on causes of death from a sampling of developed countries are shown in
Table A-3. Total annual death rates per 100,000 of population, and death rates for
the major causes of mortality (per 100,000) are also shown. These rates are not
age adjusted and must be considered in the context of the population age structures of these countries. Some of the most longevous national populations have
high mortality rates, because the populations contain relatively large proportions
of elderly people and relatively fewer young people. Thus, Sweden, a country of
high life expectancies (see Table A-1), has a high death rate, whereas the United
States has a lower death rate because of the large proportion of younger people
born during the post-World War II "baby boom." In the Swedish population
16.9% are age 65 and over, and in the United Kingdom 15.1% are 65 and over
(Torrey et al., 1987). The figures are 12.4 and 12.0% for France and the United
States, respectively, and 9.4% for Poland. In an effort to obtain comparability in
the different national data, the column on the far right of Table A-3 shows the
percentage of the total deaths attributable to each principal cause of mortality.

Inconsistencies are introduced not only by the simultaneous use of two different revisions of the *International Classification of Diseases* by different countries
but also, as discussed, by what appear to be variable national practices in completing death certificates. The category entitled "Other Circulatory Diseases" is
used to varying extents in different countries to describe vascular diseases, some
of which could surely be called ischemic heart disease. In developed countries
the category "Ill-defined Causes" is commonly used to describe 1 to 10% of
deaths, but it is used to describe fewer than 0.1% of deaths in Romania and 0.5%
of deaths in the United Kingdom.

The most frequent causes of death in the United States, ischemic heart disease,
cancer, and cerebrovascular disease, are the most common causes of death in
most but not all other developed countries. The order is different in some countries, with cancer being the most common cause of death fairly commonly, and
cerebrovascular disease being the most common cause of death in Portugal and in
some Eastern European countries. More detailed examination of data in the
*Demographic Yearbook, 1986* (United Nations, 1988) reveals large national differences in death rates from neoplasms of different organs and large differences
in death rates from accidents.

## Less-Developed Countries

Information on causes of death in the *Demographic Yearbook* (United Nations,
1988) is sparse for less-developed countries (some data are provided in Table

A-4). It must be emphasized that the data are supplied by the countries themselves to the United Nations.

Again, mortality rates must be considered in the context of population structure. The populations of these countries are young. In the Philippines, only 3.2% of the population is 65 years and older, and in Brazil the figure is 4.3% (Torrey et al., 1987). This explains low rates from the causes of death of elderly people in the developed countries—ischemic heart disease, cancer, and strokes. The infant death rate is high, as are death rates from gastroenteritis and bacilliary dysentery, which are the principal causes of infant deaths. Other infectious diseases are also seen among the most common causes of death, and accidental death is common in some countries as a reflection of the young age of much of the population as well as, perhaps, of life styles. People die from a greater variety of causes than in developed countries, and in some less-developed countries the classification "Ill-defined Causes" is used to describe up to 25% of deaths.

Although the patterns of principal causes of death are very different in these countries from those in developed countries, the pattern is not similar to that in the United States in 1900. Nowhere is tuberculosis the most common cause of death, and the other infectious diseases that have virtually disappeared in developed countries are not common causes of death in less-developed countries. Immunizations and antibiotic drugs used in their control and treatment are available worldwide and are both effective and relatively inexpensive.

## Causes of Death of Very Old People

Based on death certificate tabulations, the causes of death of Americans 85 years and older differ little from the causes of death of the United States population as a whole (National Center for Health Statistics, 1988). Ischemic heart disease, cancer, and strokes, in that order, are the three principal causes, with pneumonia, a distant fourth, at 6.5% of the total. Of the total deaths of people 85 years and over, a smaller percentage is caused by cancer and a larger percentage is caused by strokes compared with the population of all ages. The "Other Cardiovascular Diseases" category is used on a larger proportion of the death certificates of very elderly people.

The *International Classification of Diseases* (World Health Organization, 1977) provides little opportunity to designate old age as a cause of death. There is a category (290) for senile dementia, and there is a category (797) for senility without mention of psychosis, but these are little used. Senility with dementia was tabulated as a cause of 0.5% of deaths of people 85 years and older in 1986. Senility without mention of psychosis, which is part of the larger category "Signs and Symptoms, Ill-defined," was tabulated as the cause of death of less than 0.3% of those 85 years and over dying in 1986.

There is a paucity of autopsy determinations of causes of death of the very elderly. As described, 12.6% of deaths are autopsied nationally, with the rate being the highest at 55.3% for the few dying between 25 and 34 years of age. The rate is 6.9% for those dying between 65 and 74, 5.1% for those between 75 and 84, and only 2.3% for those at ages 85 and older (National Center for Health Statistics, 1988). Autopsy rates appear to be higher in the United Kingdom.

In a review of 200 autopsies on Americans 85 years and older, Kohn (1982) was unable to find an acceptable cause of death in 26% of cases. As the author stated, "Many of these persons died having aspirated gastric contents or with slight bronchopneumonia or pulmonary edema or with very small pulmonary infarcts, but no lesions or processes that would cause death in middle-aged persons were observed." The interpretation was that the persons died from "diseases and processes which have more serious consequences the older the affected person." It was suggested that, with increasing age ever smaller challenges to homeostasis can have fatal consequences. Even an autopsy examination may be unable to detect evidence that this has occurred. Pneumonia was listed as the cause of death in only 9% of cases in that study, and ischemic heart disease was the most frequently listed cause.

The results of the study by Kohn (1982) were not confirmed in a British study in which 322 autopsies on persons 65 years and older were reviewed. Although significant disagreements with death certificates were found in about one-fifth of the cases, it was impossible to find a lesion or process judged to be a cause of death in only 7.5% of persons 85 years and older (6.7% in persons aged 65 to 74) (Puxty et al., 1983). In another series of autopsies described in the same paper, a cause of death could not be found in only 4.2% of cases 85 years and older. It should be noted that the same rules that Kohn applied concerning lesions that would be designated as causes of death in younger people were applied in the British study. In the British study pneumonia was listed as the most common cause of death (30 to 40% of cases).

In a Japanese study (Ishii et al., 1980) 5,106 autopsies on persons aged 80 and older were reviewed. No indication was given that there were any cases in which a cause of death could not be determined. Although neoplasms were listed as the most frequent cause of death, pneumonia ranked second and accounted for about 30% of the deaths.

There are two American studies on the hearts of humans 90 years and older in series of consecutive autopsies (Waller and Roberts, 1983; Lie and Hammond, 1988). The results do not entirely agree, with one study showing more coronary artery disease with significant lumenal obstruction than the other, but both studies showed widespread cardiac pathology including scarring, amyloidosis, and calcification. In each study cardiovascular disease was determined to be the cause of death in fewer than half of the cases. Each study contained a case in which cause of death could not be determined. In one study pneumonia was not mentioned as a cause of death. In the other, it was included with pulmonary emboli and was determined to be the cause of death in about 30% of cases.

A recent American study of autopsies of deceased residents aged 67 to 92 of a teaching nursing home shows that during a seven-year period the autopsy rate increased from 2.4 to 10% (Gloth and Burtonk, 1990). One-third of the death certificates did not agree with reasonable interpretations of the patients' clinical records, and in only 12 of 34 cases did the certificate agree with the autopsy findings. Pneumonia was the most common cause of death (50%) as determined at autopsy, but 44% of the death certificates of the pneumonia cases did not list pneumonia as the cause of death.

An issue in these studies appears to be a variable willingness to list pneumonia as a cause of death of very elderly people, and there may be a reluctance of some American physicians to do so. Pneumonia can be the terminal event in ischemic heart disease, cancer, strokes, and other major diseases of mortality. In these cases, the underlying disease should be listed as the cause of death. Pneumonia can be one of the classic patterns, in which case it should be listed as the primary cause of death. In many cases, however, minimal inflammatory change is seen in the lungs, with coexistent aspirated gastric contents and mucous and with edema fluid consequent on heart failure. These cases may be considered cardiopulmon- ary failure, but failure is not an acceptable entry on death certificates, and some etiological entity from the *International Classification* will have to be entered to explain the failure, even if evidence for this entity is not very strong. Pneumonia is such an acceptable entity.

There is uncertainty as to the extent of pneumonia that can fairly be said to cause death, even in middle-aged people. Standard procedures for sampling lungs at autopsy to determine the extent of pneumonia do not exist. Given the heterogeneity of the very elderly population, criteria must be established to correlate pulmonary findings with the function of other organs. In view of the infrequency with which autopsies are done on very elderly people, the necessary information will be a long time in coming.

Senile dementia poses a problem of much current interest concerning the causes of death of very elderly people. The conditions of senile dementia includ- ing Alzheimer's disease, multi-infarct dementia, and Parkinson's disease occur with increasing frequency with age, and by some estimates (e.g., Evans et al., 1989) affect up to half of people 85 years and older. As stated, senile dementia seldom appears in tabulations of causes of death of the elderly, although it is recognized as life shortening (e.g., Nielsen et al., 1977). Loss of immune func- tion and difficulty swallowing are associated with senile dementia and could predispose to terminal pneumonia and other forms of infectious diseases. Too little is known, however, about why these people actually die, and mortality tabulations reflect neither the underlying condition nor the terminal pathology.

In a study from Great Britain (Burns et al., 1990), bronchopneumonia was the most frequent cause of death of persons with Alzheimer's disease, diagnosed clinically and as reflected on the death certificate and at autopsy (64%). It must be recognized that this study comes from a country where pneumonia is described much more frequently as a cause of death than in the United States. Death certificates and autopsy reports agreed as to the cause of death in 77% of cases. Senile dementia was not mentioned on the death certificate in 30% of cases. A plea is made that death certificates list dementia when there is clinical evidence for it, to provide a more accurate indication of the frequency of this condition.

Consideration of the causes of death of very old people raises profound questions. Is there such a thing as mortality in the absence of underlying fatal disease or trauma? How should multiple disease processes be evaluated in determining a final cause of death? Can functional decrements progress with age to the point that life can no longer be sustained? How should the terminal failure of vital systems be classified? Should death certificates or the *International Classification of Disease* be altered to reflect functional decrements of very old people, or is this encouraging laziness? If longevity is usually determined by the course of late life diseases, then is human senescence simply an increasing predisposition to these diseases? Are the genes controlling longevity simply genes for disease resistance? What about animals with different life spans and different causes of death? Is there any determinant of longevity that applies to many kinds of living things?

## Causes of Death of Lower Animals

As described in Chapter 1, most living things have finite life spans that are characteristic for each species, but that range widely if all animal species are considered collectively. In this chapter it has been emphasized that there are a few clearly defined causes of mortality for most humans in developed countries. These are diseases that usually occur at advanced ages, making them common in societies in which causes of human mortality at younger ages have been largely eliminated. What are the principal causes of death of animals when they are kept under carefully controlled conditions so that their survival curves are shaped much like those of humans in developed countries (see curve C in Fig. 1-1 and the most recent American survival curves, Fig. 1-2)? Are there any lessons to be learned about human mortality by considering the principal causes of death of animals?

Fruit flies (*Drosophila melanogaster*), a favorite experimental animal in gerontological research, go through larval and pupal stages and live a few tens of days as adults. There are genetic strains with unusually short life spans as adults and more significantly, strains with unusually long life spans (Luckinbill and Clare, 1985; Rose and Graves, 1989). Although there is no certain answer to the question of the major causes of death of fruit flies, something is known about the pathology with which and probably of which they die. A significant finding in senescent fruit flies is the cessation of digestive tract function, with the postmito-tic cells lining the digestive tract accumulating lipofuscin pigment, which is derived from membrane breakdown. The neurons of the minimal nervous system that has little redundancy gradually drop out late in life. Old flies die constipated and largely immobilized.

Another well-studied invertebrate of much current interest to gerontologists is the nematode *Caenorhabditis elegans*. The embryonic derivation of every one of its approximately 1,000 somatic cells is understood, and, with the exception of the gonads, it also is composed of postmitotic cells. There is a long-lived mutant that has a mean and a maximum life span 70 and 110% longer, respectively, than the parental strains (Friedman and Johnson, 1988a and b). As with fruit flies, these organisms cease moving and feeding as they grow older, and eventually the digestive tract breaks down, permitting invasion by bacteria.

An important difference between these invertebrates and mammals is that the cells in most mammalian tissues, including the digestive system, are capable of replacement through cell division. Some mammalian organs, however, also con-tain postmitotic cells that cannot be replaced, including the muscle cells of the heart and the neurons of the central nervous system, as described previously. It is true that even during human life these irreplaceable cells slowly die (Martin, 1977a). Most human mortality, in fact, results from functional failure in the heart and brain, and one may wonder whether nematodes and fruit flies are a model of mortality resulting from the loss of postmitotic cells. An important difference is that most human death results not from the gradual dropping out of postmitotic cells, but from the acute massive death of such cells as a result of ischemia consequent on the obstruction of blood vessels. Fruit flies and nematodes have no heart or circulatory system, and it is unlikely that their cell death is based on ischemia.

Laboratory rodents have hearts and circulatory systems and cellular prolifera-tive capabilities within organs that are similar to those of humans. Their mainte-nance under laboratory conditions, including some strains that are kept under pathogen-free conditions, is perhaps most analogous to the condition of humans living in developed societies.

In several rat studies the most common pathological lesion consistent with mortality is nephrosclerosis or chronic glomerulopathy (Bolton et al., 1976; Coleman et al., 1977; Anver et al., 1982; Gray et al., 1982; Maeda et al., 1985;

Yu et al., 1985). These renal lesions include occlusion of the capillaries of the glomeruli, thickening of the glomerular basement membranes, and atrophy of the tubules. If the severity and extent of the pathology are graded on a scale of 0 to $5^+$, the lesions are more severe in older rats. The more severe lesions result in renal dysfunction, including the retention of blood urea nitrogen and serum creatinine and urinary loss of albumin. Probably homeostasis breaks down and death occurs quickly in the more severely affected animals. The lesions do not appear to be ischemic in their pathogenesis. Immune complexes are found in the glomeruli, but in the absence of components of complement, it cannot be said that the pathogenesis of nephrosclerosis is inflammatory.

Renal function deteriorates slowly with age in humans (Lindeman, 1981), and lesions that gradually appear do not differ much from those of rodent nephrosclerosis (Smith et al., 1989). The functional decrements, however, do not usually affect the requirements for homeostasis. The functional reserve of human kidneys is in excess of the required minimum by four- or fivefold early in life, and renal failure is not a major cause of human death. The schedule of renal aging in humans seems to be slower than the schedule of renal aging in rats relative to life span, and the functional reserve of the human kidneys far outlasts the more disease-prone cardiovascular system.

Myocarditis, inflammation in the cardiac muscle, is common in older rats, but it appears not to be of ischemic origin. One looks in vain for ischemic heart disease and cerebrovascular disease in laboratory rodents, and these animals are resistant to atherosclerosis even on atherogenic diets.

There are also differences between the malignant tumors commonly causing death in humans and in laboratory rodents. Rodent tumors are very strain specific and commonly associated with viruses. Although malignant lymphomas and mammary carcinomas are found in both humans and some strains of laboratory rodents, the carcinomas of the bronchi, stomach, colon, and female genitalia, which are common causes of human death, are of rare occurrence in rodents (Wolf et al., 1988), and, in fact, in other animals, such as cats and dogs, which are commonly allowed to live out their natural life spans.

Primate pathology has been studied extensively, and most of the lesions found in humans have also been found in various primate species, including atherosclerosis, myocardial infarction, and the common human neoplasms (Fiennes, 1972). Autopsies of macaques dying in large colonies, however, reveal very different incidences of diseases and causes of death than in humans. In 370 consecutive autopsies of rhesus monkeys in the Yerkes colony, the most common causes of death were pulmonary ascariasis (caused by a round worm), pleuritis, enterocolitis, pneumonia, and peritonitis, in that order. Neoplasms were found in only 14 of the 370 autopsies. Not a single cardiac death was recorded (McClure, 1975a; 1975b). In a study of free-ranging rhesus monkeys, tetanus caused 25 percent of all mortality (Kessler and Rawlins, 1984). In another study (Baba et al., 1979) both coronary atherosclerosis and cardiac fibrosis presumably related to ischemia were described, but it is stated that they were less common and less advanced than in humans.

Therefore, even today most captive primates under the best of conditions die of infectious diseases, which could be controlled and treated and much reduced in frequency and as causes of death. What will be causes of death if infectious diseases are better controlled? Will primates in captivity live longer? Will zoo records of maximum species longevity become even longer? What might Table 1-1 look like some time in the future when infectious diseases are no longer major causes of death of primates in captivity? In comparing human and nonhuman primate longevity, it must be remembered that even centuries ago when infectious diseases were the usual causes of human mortality, there were humans living into their 80s, and possibly longer. They may have been outlyers with special resistance to the infectious diseases, or they may have had less exposure to these diseases. If, in fact, nonhuman primates have much greater longevities than present records indicate, one would expect to see occasional individuals in captivity today living close to the maximum species longevity.

Will ischemic heart disease and cerebrovascular disease become major causes of death of nonhuman primates? Probably not unless the animals are fed atherogenic diets with about 40 percent of calories as fat, comparable to human diets in the United States. These diets are atherogenic in only some species. In other species there are individuals known as "responders" that become hypercholesterolemic on atherogenic diets (Vesselinovich, 1988). The feedback relationship between dietary cholesterol and hepatic cholesterol synthesis seems not to function in these individuals. The arterial lesions seen in these hypercholesterolemic animals on atherogenic diets depend on rates of cholesterol deposition and vary from fatty streaks in the aortas of rabbits to complex atheromatous plaques in the aortas of pigs and some nonhuman primates. Many animal species and "non-responders" are virtually invulnerable to the development of atherosclerosis by any dietary manipulation.

## Conclusions

Increased longevity in developed countries is consistent with the changing causes of death. The causes of death of young people of the past have largely disappeared. People live longer. They still die, but of causes that seldom affect young people. Causes of death of the very old are sometimes more obscure and appear not to involve the major diseases of mortality. In less-developed countries one can also observe changing causes of death as infectious diseases are conquered and more people reach advanced ages. Populations in less-developed countries show various stages in approaching the longevity pattern of developed countries.

Causes of death of animals up to the level of nonhuman primates are different from causes of human death. The most striking contrast is the importance of atherosclerosis and its ischemic consequences, which is involved in most human mortality, but which is uncommon in other species, and there are other differences. One may ask how universal is mortality as a process when the routes to it vary so widely in different species? The question has no present answer, but it is raised here in the context of biomedical determinants of longevity, which is the topic of the next chapter.

# 3

# Biomedical Determinants of Longevity

in mortal flesh we hold our frail abode.

PHILLIP DODDRIDGE (1702–1751)
English preacher, poet and hymnist
From a verse to which many hymn tunes have been adapted

The life span of each individual results from interactions of many biomedical factors. Given the causes of death of humans today, the factors and their interactions are different from those operating in other animals, as well as in humans of the past. The factors considered in this chapter are diverse, with the principal unifying theme being that each has something to do with mortality. (a) Some are genetically based, with well-defined genes or at least well-defined hereditary patterns. (b) Some concern somatic maintenance—the ability to repair and replace wear and tear that accumulates during the life span. There is a literature that the "investment in somatic maintenance" (Kirkwood, 1985, 1987) is an important determinant of longevity. Mechanisms of somatic maintenance are genetically based. (c) Some suggest programs in which aging and mortality may be part of development, and such programs are genetically based and reflect changes in gene expression. These do not add up to a coherent and global explanation of life span and mortality. For this reason, the factors are considered separately.

## Genes and Life Spans

Most mutations are harmful, and mutations often directly shorten life. There are long lists of genetic diseases (McKusick, 1988), and some of these diseases cause reduced life span. Mutations result in erroneous amino acid sequences in vital protein molecules, that may manifest aberrations such as reduced enzyme activity and increased lability. Mutations may also result in aberrations in gene expression, such as in the amount of molecules synthesized. The qualitative and quantitative hemoglobinopathies (Honig and Adams, 1986) are good examples of such mutations, although these diseases are not major causes of death. Not all amino acid substitutions in hemoglobin or other proteins result in molecules with altered properties that cause diseases, but many do.

Some life-shortening mutations are recognized today only as base changes in DNA or as gene products (proteins) of uncertain function and of questionable application to the associated disease, for example, the recently described gene for cystic fibrosis (Estivil et al., 1989; Ianuzzi et al., 1989). This mutant gene was recognized from restriction fragment polymorphisms (RFLP's) affecting a gene complex of no known function. The more recent isolation of a gene product of the cystic fibrosis gene has yielded a mutant protein that seems to reduce cellular responses to cyclic AMP (Baringa, 1992). This may or may not explain the inability to export chloride in diseased cells, and it does not explain other features of this life-shortening disease.

An interesting approach to longevity-limiting alleles has been taken by George Martin (1978), who examined the catalog of hereditary diseases (McKusick, 1975) and found that about 7 percent of the conditions manifest some aspect of what he called an aging phenotype. Considering that not all of the aging phenotype characteristics involve the shortening of life (e.g., graying and thinning of the hair), and that many of the hereditary diseases manifesting an aspect of the aging phenotype are not characterized by life shortening, only a few genes may commonly limit the human life span.

Genes that extend life are more difficult to recognize. They may be genes that confer resistance to the common diseases of mortality. If the death of people at advanced ages has less to do with easily recognized diseases, life prolongation genes may reduce the progress of late life functional decrements and, thus, increase the capacity to compensate for challenges to homeostasis. Alternatively, they may increase processes of repair and replacement of vital structures and correct damage resulting from the wear and tear of passing time. Genes that may extend the maximum human life span are discussed in Chapter 6 in the context of the evolution of longevity.

## Correlations with Animal Longevity

As shown in Table 1-1, the maximum life spans of mammalian species range over a factor of 100 or more. No matter how well they are maintained, mice, dogs, and horses will not live as long, on average, as humans. Biological factors that may correlate with species life spans have been researched. Correlations with body weights and more specifically with brain weight (encephalization), as described in Chapter 1, are too complex to be of use in considering specific processes that could affect species survival under controlled conditions. These correlations will be discussed in Chapter 6 in the context of the evolution of longevity in primates. The correlations between longevity and DNA repair and other genes of uncertain function are discussed in this chapter.

## DNA Repair and Longevity

A striking and potentially useful correlation has been described between the maximum life spans of several mammalian species and a type of DNA repair activity. The observation that this DNA repair is more active in the human species than in shorter lived mammals suggests some relationship with longevity.

DNA is only one of the macromolecules damaged during the life span, but it is the most irreplaceable of all molecular targets. Each cell contains only two chromosomes, of each kind, and each chromosome contains only one DNA double helical strand representing each gene and its complement. DNA contains the information for the synthesis and accumulation of everything else in the cell, and the distribution of the information to daughter cells requires the intactness of each DNA molecule. DNA damage occurs as a result of reactions between DNA and reactive chemical groups and from the effects of ionizing radiations. Damage to the DNA results in cross-linked DNA strands, which cannot be replicated and divided as required for cell division, and in altered bases, which pass on somatic mutations to somatic daughter cells. If germ cells are affected, then mutations are passed to future generations.

It was first shown by Hart and Setlow (1974) that the excision repair of DNA damaged by ultraviolet light is more active in longer lived species. Several biochemical steps are required in excision repair, including recognition of the damage, excision of DNA in the region of the damage, replacement of the excised DNA, and closure of the break when the replacement is complete (Friedberg, 1985). What actually was measured in these studies was the incorporation of a pyrimidine deoxyribose nucleoside (the DNA building block, thymidine) into the nuclei of ultraviolet light-irradiated cultured skin fibroblasts. The measurements of repair activity were by autoradiography, and the process observed is described as "unscheduled DNA synthesis," because the incorporation of thymidine was observed in the presence of an inhibitor that blocks DNA synthesis for cell replication but not DNA synthesis for repair. Ultraviolet light causes several kinds of DNA damage (Friedberg, 1985), and it is not known what types of DNA lesions were repaired and which step of the DNA repair reactions was limiting. It is, therefore, not known what genes are involved.

The original observation by Hart and Setlow (1974) was of seven species from five mammalian orders with approximately a 50-fold range of maximum life spans, from shrews to humans. The repair activity observed had a 10-fold range of initial rates and a sixfold range in the amount of thymidine incorporated in completed reactions.

The observation has been expanded in other investigations. The correlation between the activity in excision repair of ultraviolet-damaged DNA and maximum species life span was observed in the fibroblasts of two mouse species, *Mus musculus* and *Peromyscus leucopus*, which have a two- to threefold difference in maximum life spans (Hart et al., 1979). The correlation was noted in comparing DNA repair in the embryonic fibroblasts of three inbred mouse strains with different maximum life spans (Paffenholz, 1978) and also in both the fibroblasts and lymphocytes of several primate species (Hall et al., 1984; Bowden, 1979).

Kato and colleagues (1980) found some exceptions to the correlation. Although the same relative values were seen in animals that had been studied by other workers, studies of other species representing 11 mammalian orders showed little correlation, with important exceptions being found among bats and shorter lived primates (Tice and Setlow, 1985).

One may wonder about the significance of the repair of ultraviolet DNA damage to longevity. Only cells within the first millimeter or two of the body surface are exposed to ultraviolet light, and death rarely occurs because of these cells. It can even be questioned how much human death can be attributed to unrepaired DNA damage of any kind anywhere in the body. Evidence for age-related accumulation of DNA damage in humans is not impressive (Tice and Setlow, 1985). On the other hand, it has been shown that rat cells accumulate high levels of unrepaired oxidative DNA damage. This damage causes mutations that may contribute to the short life spans and the high incidence of tumors in these animals (Ames and Gold, 1991). Thus, although the correlation of life span and the repair of DNA ultraviolet damage is of uncertain significance today, it is close enough to basic molecular processes to be of continuing interest, and it could be indicative of other aspects of DNA repair or of genomic plasticity in ways that are not recognized today. Somatic maintenance includes the repair of DNA damage, and longer lived species should have a greater investment in somatic maintenance.

*Correlation of Genes of Uncertain Function with Longevity*

The laboratory of Edmond Yunis has taken a very different approach to correlating genetic content to longevity (Yunis et al., 1988). They studied the base sequences of DNA segments in mouse strains that showed variations in the length of survival (mean and maximum) over a twofold range. Each strain was typed using markers of 141 genetic regions located on 15 chromosomes, and several correlations were found. The precise genes and their functions remain unknown, and the large number of genetic markers that correlate with survival is surprising. The mechanisms favoring survival may include resistance to specific causes of death and more effective repair of damage to vital molecules as well as possible involvement of some genes in a larger program of development that includes conditions of senescence that predispose to mortality.

In some ways this research has its counterpart in the research on the genes associated with cystic fibrosis already mentioned, except that in this case DNA was defined as associated with characteristic life spans rather than with a life-shortening disease.

## Heredity and Human Longevity

It has long been believed that heredity has something to do with human longevity: "If ye would live long, choose well thy ancestors." The issue has been the subject of many investigations over the years, based on family pedigrees, insurance records, and both parents and offspring of long-lived individuals. Generally modest correlations have been found that indicate a familial component to longevity (Cohen, 1964; Murphy, 1978).

Some problems are inherent in the investigations that have been done and include the following:

1. Familial correlations are not necessarily based on genetics. Clearly social and environmental factors have strong familial components that may affect life spans, generally in the direction of increasing the apparent similarity of family members.
2. Changes in causes of death during the past century (see Chapter 2) must be associated with changing genetic factors conferring resistance and susceptibility. For example, it has long been suspected that there are genetic factors affecting resistance and susceptibility to tuberculosis, although little is known about what these factors may be. This topic resurfaces fairly frequently, often in the context of racial differences in susceptibility (e.g., Stead et al., 1990). Such factors would have been very important determinants of longevity in the first years of this century when tuberculosis was a common cause of death, but they are quite unimportant in America today. On the other hand, genes affecting cholesterol levels are much more important as contemporary determinants of longevity. Intergenerational patterns of longevity are affected by changes in the causes of death.

The problem of intergenerational comparisons is obviated by studies on twins, which also control for social and environmental factors. Twin studies offer the opportunity to compare monozygotic twins who have identical genotypes and dizygotic twins who are no more closely related than other siblings. A formula[1] has been developed to estimate the inherited contributions of a characteristic for which monozygotic and dizygotic twins are compared. Studies of monozygotic twins show impressive correlations in longevity and have given major clues to genetic determinants of longevity (Bank and Jarvik, 1978; Goldbourt and Neufeld, 1986).

The study of sibling adoptees raised in different homes offers a way of distinguishing genetic and environmental effects. A paper from Denmark (Sorenson et al., 1988) showed strong correlations between parental death at ages less than 50 years and the early death of adoptees from infectious and cardiovascular diseases. The correlations were not strong between parental death over age 70 and longer lives of the adoptees. The absence of a correlation in cancer deaths suggests that environmental factors predominate over genetic factors in its etiology.

## Familial Risk Factors in the Major Causes of Human Death

Clearly, genetics affecting the risk factors for the major causes of death of humans in economically developed societies constitute major biomedical determinants of longevity. As mentioned in Chapter 2 and elaborated here, some well-defined familial and, in some cases, genetic contributions to the risk factors are recognized.

### Vascular Diseases

Genetics are a major determinant of life span as related to ischemic heart disease, with recognized alleles leading to early death from this cause and to phenotypes that are consistent with long life. The risk of death from myocardial infarction is increased 1.5- to twofold in a man whose male sibling died at an early age (less than 50 years) from this cause. Among monozygotic twins, the concordance rate is greater than 50 percent in death from myocardial infarction.

Ethnic differences in death rates from myocardial infarction appear to result more from genetic than, for example, from dietary factors. This was seen in Israeli Jews of various origins and in age-adjusted death rates from coronary heart disease among Japanese and Americans or persons from Western European countries (Goldbourt and Neufeld, 1986). On the other hand, studies on Japanese in Japan, people of Japanese descent in Hawaii, and in mainland United States (see Chapter 4) indicate that nongenetic factors also play a major role in the

---

1. Heritability = 2(Concordance rate in monozygotic twins − Concordance rate in dizygotic twins).

incidence of coronary heart disease, which differs greatly in incidence in these three populations.

One study shows that restriction fragment length polymorphisms (RFLPs) in cases of early death from myocardial infarction are associated with hyper-cholesterolemia, although the functions of the genes encoded by the DNA in the fragments are not known (Price et al., 1989). Another study found variations in the apolipoprotein B (see Chapter 2) gene that was associated with obesity, high blood cholesterol levels, and increased risk of coronary heart disease (Rajput-Williams et al., 1988).

Only a few cases of hyperlipidemia can be attributed to monogenic conditions (Segal et al., 1982; Goldbourt and Neufeld, 1986) and the best defined is familial hypercholesterolemia (Ose and Tolleshaug, 1989). In this condition the low-density lipoproteins (LDLs) are elevated because of defects (several alleles are recognized) in the LDL receptor protein, which is needed for the removal of LDLs from the circulation to sites such as endocrine organs, where the choles-terol steroid structure is used for hormone synthesis. Hypercholesterolemia is aggravated by low intracellular cholesterol levels, therefore the feedback inhibi-tion of cholesterol synthesis is reduced. About 1 in 200 to 300 persons are heterozygous for this disorder, and even the heterozygotes usually die at early ages from ischemic heart disease. Familial hypercholesterolemia must be re-garded as a life-shortening genetic disease.

Rare conditions in which LDLs are low or absent because apoprotein B is deficient might appear to be advantageous to longevity. There is hypo-cholesterolemia in some of these cases; however, clinical disorders coexist that can be attributed to low cellular and biliary cholesterol, including malfunction of the central nervous system and deficient absorption of fat-soluble vitamins (Segal et al., 1982).

Familial deficiencies have been found in the apoproteins A-1 that lead to low levels of the high-density lipoproteins (HDLs) and the early development of atherosclerosis. There are conditions with elevated levels of the very low-density lipoproteins (VLDLs) that contain triglycerides, elevated levels of which are also a risk factor in the early development of atherosclerosis.

Diabetes is a risk factor in both ischemic heart disease and in cerebrovascular disease. Diabetes leads to vascular pathology, including atherosclerosis and dis-ease in smaller vessels. Both the insulin-dependent diabetes of younger people and the insulin-independent diabetes (type II) found characteristically in older adults have genetic components. In the case of insulin-dependent diabetes, there is evidence of mutations in the gene for insulin and in the promotor sequence of that gene. In the case of type II diabetes there is evidence of mutations in the gene for the insulin receptor (Shimada et al., 1990) and in enzymes of sugar metabolism.

Hypertension, another risk factor in ischemic heart disease and in cerebrovascular disease, also has a genetic component with striking ethnic and familial aggregations. The gene or genes involved in human hypertension are unknown, but in hereditary rat hypertension there is evidence of a mutation of the gene in renin, a hormone with an effect on vascular tone that is elaborated by the kidney in response to adrenal mineralocorticoid hormones (Leckie, 1992).

Given the high percentage of deaths from vascular diseases and the large genetic components involved in pathogenesis, it is surprising that evidence for familial influences on life span is not more striking. As time passes and successive generations die of ischemic heart disease and cerebrovascular disease, it is likely that intergenerational evidence of inherited life span will become more impressive.

### Cancer

Most cancer occurs sporadically without much evidence of familial clustering. In most cases, a lifetime exposure to carcinogens seems to be more important than any hereditary predisposition. There are families, called "cancer families," with high incidence of the same tumor, for example, female breast cancer. There is also evidence for the inheritance of some less common cancers (Hansen and Cavenel, 1987; Li, 1988).

Several genetic mechanisms are recognized that could be operative in cancer susceptibility and resistance and would affect cancer incidence and the time of its appearance. In the case of familial breast cancer, a mutant gene has been recognized (Faust and Meeker, 1992), although the function of this gene remains uncertain. Expression of the allele is estrogen inducible. Mutations that inactivate p53, a tumor suppressor gene (Sager, 1989), have been found in some cases of several kinds of cancer. Conformational changes and post-translational modifications in the p53 protein have been invoked as other kinds of changes that could permit the proliferation of cancer cells (Ulrich et al., 1992). In other investigations, mutations affecting base sequences and expression of oncogenes have been described (e.g., Rodenhuis and Slebos, 1992). Chromosomal translocations have also been recognized in some tumors. These genetic changes could be somatic, as part of a multistep process of carcinogenesis involving the progenitor cell of the tumor, or could be transmitted from generation to generation through germ cells. Genes involved in the metabolism of environmental carcinogenic chemicals to ultimate carcinogens could also affect cancer.

### Immune Function

Diminished immune function with age has been observed in humans and in experimental animals (Hausman and Weksler, 1985; Miller, 1990). There is much scatter in the data and much overlap between results obtained with older and younger subjects. Measurements of immune function vary on a short-term basis, making both longitudinal and cross sectional studies difficult. Still, the trend seems to be a decline in several parameters of immune competence with age. There is considerable agreement on the following generalizations:

1. The response to mitogenic stimulation of T lymphocytes diminishes with age.
2. The production of the lymphokine interleukin-2 (Il-2), the ultimate T-lymphocyte mitogen, falls off with age.
3. The response of T lymphocytes to Il-2 declines with age.
4. The ability of B lymphocytes to respond to antigenic stimulation diminishes with age. Inasmuch as B-lymphocyte function is dependent on T lymphocytes, it is not certain whether this is a primary or a secondary effect, or both.
5. There is an increased tendency of B lymphocytes to respond inappropriately to antigenic stimulation with age, with the more frequent production of autoantibodies.

The mechanisms of these changes are not known, and studies are indicative of the complexity of the immune system. It appears that smaller proportions of cell populations are responsive in later life, and more attention must be given to subpopulations of the helper, killer, and uncommitted T lymphocytes. Studies of the T-lymphocyte responses to mitogens suggest that the intracellular response to mitogenic stimulation in the form of increased intracellular ionized calcium is reduced with age, but this could represent a change in cell population rather than a change in cellular responsiveness (Miller, 1991).

The increasing incidences of cancer and infectious diseases in elderly people are often attributed to declining levels of immune function. It is well recognized that antibody responses, such as to influenza vaccine, are reduced in elderly people (Ershler et al., 1985), and this has an obvious effect on survival. Autoantibodies are commonly found in the elderly, but these are usually not associated with autoimmune diseases, which have their peak incidence in younger adults.

Two studies showed that stronger immune function in elderly people is a predictor of longevity (Roberts-Thomson et al., 1974; Murasko et al., 1988). In each case the measurements were chiefly of T-lymphocyte function. The findings are puzzling in that most of the elderly subjects died from heart disease and cerebrovascular disease, which have no recognized association with immune function. It is not completely ruled out that some of the subjects with less immune competence were sick at the beginning of the studies and that the reduced immune function was a consequence of preexistent disease, which was the cause of death. Another possibility is that reduced immune function is a biomarker of aging and is indicative of reduced biological fitness that precedes death—actually a biomarker of mortality. It may be a component of reduced fitness without being causally related to mortality in every case.

The concept of biomarkers of aging has been discussed extensively (Baker and Sprott, 1988), and there is a search for markers that may be so basic and so widespread as to indicate a general process underlying aging, resulting in some of its features, and leading to mortality. Changes in immune function remain an important topic in the investigation of the biomedical determinants of longevity.

## Histocompatibility Antigens

The system of histocompatibility antigens, designated HLA in humans, determines the antigenic characteristics of cell surfaces, which are important in the recognition of self in immune tolerance and in graft and transplant rejection or acceptance. The system is under the control of several gene loci (different genes in different locations in the genome) and of multiple alleles (alternative mutant genes) at each locus. The loci and alleles are variable in their expression in different individuals and in different kinds of cells. A system of histocompatibility antigens in mice, designated H-2, discussed at the end of this section, has many parallels to the human HLA system.

Given the diversity of loci, alleles, and expression, there is much polymorphism of histocompatibility. HLA characteristics, being hereditary, have familial, geographic, and ethnic correlations. Many statistically significant correlations have been found between HLA types and clinical conditions (Tiwari and Terasaki, 1985; Thomson, 1988). There are large differences in relative risk of these diseases in various ethnically defined populations. Although most of the striking correlations have been shown with rheumatoid diseases, which are believed to have autoimmune components, correlations have also been found with infectious diseases, malignant tumors, psychiatric diseases, and some conditions that are not readily classified. Some of the correlations probably reflect aberrant immunological functions resulting in pathogenic processes such as inflammation and cell killing. Sometimes viral infection and hapten binding appear to set off autoimmunity that has disease-related predispositions based on histocompatibility. Some correlations appear to be the result of genetic linkage between HLA loci and nearby genes that have roles in pathogenesis. Some of the correlations with disease involve life-threatening and life-shortening conditions, whereas others involve conditions of morbidity and disability without major effects on survival.

Although most of the correlations observed are between HLA alleles and clinical conditions, a recent study described a correlation between an HLA allele and longevity (Takata et al., 1987; Editorial, *Lancet*, 1987). A comparison of 80 HLA phenotypes in nonagenarian and centenarian Okinawan Japanese and a control population of younger Okinawan Japanese revealed two significant correlations: (a) the frequency of the phenotype DRw9 was five times higher in the control population than in the very old subjects. DRw9 is found in approximately half of Orientals with a variety of diseases with autoimmune components, including systemic lupus erythematosis, insulin-dependent diabetes mellitus, and ulcerative colitis, whereas it occurs in only about 20% of Orientals without these diseases. (b) DR1, a very rare phenotype among the controls, was found in 10% of the nonagenarians and 6.7% of the centenarians. The correlations suggest that just as DRw9 seems to be a deleterious allele, DR1 may confer some advantage—at least the advantage of no predisposition to a disease or process that shortens life. Enigmatically, DR1 has been described as a risk factor in the development of thyroid cancer in Italians (Tiwari and Terasaki, 1985).

About 10 years before the study on Japanese Okinawans, Walford and his group described correlations between maximum life spans and H-2 alleles in congenic mouse strains (Smith and Walford, 1977). Correlations were found with life spans, and interestingly, a strong correlation was also found between the H-2 allele associated with the greatest life span and the strongest mitogenic response to the mitogen phytohemagglutinin. No correlation was found between mitogenic response and the allele associated with the shortest life span. Because the response to mitogens is an aspect of the immune response, one may wonder if this is evidence that the strength of the immune response is a major determinant of life span.

## The Neuroendocrine System:
## Programmed Involution and Senescence

Reproductive senescence is an event that occurs well short of the maximum life span in many species. In humans and laboratory rodents reproductive senescence occurs about halfway between birth and the maximum species life span, as discussed in Chapter 6. It occurs at about the same age and involves the same events in all individuals of the same sex of a species. Included are neuroendocrine changes, changes in the gonads, and changes in secondary sexual structures such as the breasts. These changes must be considered involutional. There are far-reaching effects on other tissues that are influenced by sex hormones, such as skin, muscle, and bone, and reproductive senescence changes the metabolism and transport of cholesterol (see Chapter 5). Reproductive senescence is an important aspect of the aging phenotype in humans, even if the actual changes contribute little to mortality.

In female mammals the basis of reproductive senescence is the disappearance of germ cells from the ovaries (Finch, 1987; Meites et al., 1987), with a consequent cessation of gamete (ovum) production and the production of estrogenic and progesteroid hormones, which come from the ovarian follicles. After reproductive senescence these hormones decrease to levels found after castration of younger animals. The process of reproductive senescence in women occurs during a brief period called menopause. It occurs more gradually in men, with the production of sperm sometimes continuing into the 70s and beyond. Moreover, the production of male steroid sex hormones by the testis is not dependent on sperm production and continues to a more advanced age than the production of sex hormones in women.

Questions concerning reproductive senescence include the following:

1. What changes lead to reproductive senescence? What is the program that controls this process so that it occurs at a relatively fixed point in the life span? Could it be genetically encoded?
2. Are the changes of reproductive senescence coordinated with other changes that lead to aging and ultimately to death?

It is unlikely that the administration of sex hormones could prolong the maximum human life span, but it does postpone some of the effects of hormone deficiency. This is the basis for the administration of estrogens to postmenopausal women to retard bone demineralization. Recognizing the risks and morbidity of the hip and vertebral fractures of osteoporosis, this is an example of the beneficial effects of hormone replacement. Estrogen replacement also has beneficial effects in the transport of cholesterol (see Chapter 5). Its negative effects include an increase in blood coagulability and the stimulation of growth of some breast cancer cells.

The immune system is subject to neuroendocrine influences, with the most clear cut being the moderation of immune responses by glucocorticoids secreted by the adrenal cortex, which is under the control of the pituitary gland. At present, there is little evidence that the age-related decrements in human immune function result from increased glucocorticoid secretion (Munck et al., 1984).

There is no evidence, in fact, that adrenal hypercorticism exists in humans in late life, however, it is important in the mortality of some other species such as the Pacific salmon.

Thus, the importance of the neuroendocrine system to mortality remains uncertain, but there are some gerontologists (e.g., Dilman, 1981) who believe that the changes of aging are in large measure programmed into the neuroendocrine system, and that the changes leading to morbidity and mortality result from the programmed malfunction of the neuroendocrine system.

## Programmed Cell Death

Programmed cell death (also called apoptosis) is a part of the developmental process. A good example is the disappearance of the tail of the tadpole, and there are many instances of programmed cell death in human development such as the regression of the vestigial urogenital structures, of the thymus, and of the deciduous teeth. The involutional changes of reproductive senescence involve the death of cells dependent on hormones. Some consider the turnover of blood cells and the cells of epithelial surfaces as programmed cell death (Gerschenson and Rotello, 1992). Those who would look for common features in the many instances of programmed cell death point out the lack of inflammation in contrast to cell death by hypoxia and by viral killing. There is often evidence of gene action, with inhibitors of transcription and translation inhibiting programmed cell death.

There is a great diversity of mechanisms triggering programmed cell killing including withdrawal of trophic requirements, influx of calcium, glucocorticoid toxicity, ubiquitin tagging of major protein constituents, and cytokine activity (Fesus et al., 1991; Whitfield, 1992).

A question is whether programmed cell death ever plays a role in decrements in function in elderly humans. Is the death of the individual a programmed event if some fatal disease does not intervene first?

## Macromolecular Damage

During the life span there is wear and tear that affects molecules. Theories of aging differ as to the importance of exogenous damage and endogenous damage (Hayflick, 1985; Cristofalo, 1988). DNA damage and repair have been discussed.

Proteins are also subject to wear and tear, with amidation, cross-linking, and oxidation being well-recognized reactions that alter the properties of proteins (Stadtman, 1988; Lee and Cerami, 1990). Many studies show the accumulation of enzyme molecules of decreased enzymatic activity in older organisms. The turnover of these molecules is reduced.

Collagen, the extracellular product of fibroblasts, accumulates with age, replacing parenchymal cells and thickening the walls of blood vessels. The properties of collagen from older animals and humans are different from those of younger individuals, with collagen aging occurring earlier in short-lived animals (Harrison and Archer, 1983). The epsilon amino group of lysine, one of the principal amino acids of collagen, reacts with reducing sugars to form cross-links between collagen fibers (Cerami et al., 1987). This process is accelerated in diabetes mellitus, in which there are elevated glucose levels, with cross-linked collagen contributing to the clinical aspects of the disease. Ultraviolet light causes cross-linking of collagen fibers in the skin, as reflected in skin wrinkles in exposed areas. Cross-linking slows the turnover of collagen and favors its accumulation. The cross-linking of rat tail collagen with age is well defined; however, the extent of cross-linking does not correlate with the life spans of individual rats (Harrison and Archer, 1983). It is a biomarker of aging without being a biomarker of mortality in these animals.

Membrane lipids are subject to peroxidation by oxidizing radicals and accumulate as intracellular lipid-rich deposits called lipofuscin (Donato and Sohal, 1981), especially in postmitotic cells. The deposits may accumulate to the extent of 5 to 10 percent of the cellular volume compromising cell function and contributing to cell death.

There are storage forms of iron that accumulate in cells with age and give rise to oxidizing radicals (Halliwell, 1987). Aging has some characteristics of a "storage disease" in that cells accumulate inert and even deleterious material that results from wear and tear.

The prevention and repair of protein damage is not as well defined as the repair of DNA damage. Some of it involves the scavenging of oxidizing radicals. A correlation has been observed between species life spans and the enzyme superoxide dismutase, which destroys oxidizing radicals, although the correlation is less impressive than the correlation between life spans and the repair of ultraviolet DNA damage (Tolmasoff et al., 1980). Interestingly, at least in mice, there are genes affecting the activity of superoxide dismutase that are linked to histocompatibility loci (Novak et al., 1979).

The deleterious effects of macromolecular damage must be considered along with the mechanisms and costs of somatic maintenance (see Chapter 6) as determinants of longevity.

## Cell Proliferation

Human somatic cells in culture are generally mortal. They are capable of a finite number of divisions, and although some may live on as postmitotic cells for a substantial time, ultimately they die. This phenomenon, known as *clonal senescence*, is sometimes taken as a correlate at the cellular level of the mortality of whole organisms. It can also be regarded as an age-related decrement at the cellular level. The original observation of clonal senescence was made on fetal fibroblasts, the cells of connective tissue that synthesize collagen (Hayflick and Moorhead, 1961; Hayflick, 1965). Human fetal fibroblasts are capable of about 50 doublings, and clonal senescence has since been observed in many other cell lines with different numbers of doublings before a limit is reached (Martin, 1977b). There remains a question about some blood cell precursors that are capable of many more divisions or that may not show clonal senescence (Harrison et al., 1984). Fewer divisions occur in cells from cases of progeria and Werner's disease, which are human diseases characterized by premature aging (appearance of an aged phenotype) and life shortening (Martin et al., 1970).

Cancer cells are immortal. Cells taken from malignant tumors or cells transformed in culture with tumor viruses or carcinogenic chemicals and that develop into malignant tumors on transplantation into suitable host animals multiply indefinitely in culture. Some tumor cell lines have been maintained for decades in culture, with approximately daily doublings. Significantly, the number of chromosomes is greater in these cells and in malignant tumors generally than in non-neoplastic cells.

Clonal senescence seems to be under genetic control, which disappears in neoplastic transformation. In somatic hybrids (heterokaryons) with a nucleus each from a mortal somatic cell and an immortal tumor cell, clonal senescence is dominant (Ning and Pereira-Smith, 1991). The hybrid cell with both nuclei undergoes clonal senescence. Only a few genes are involved in the difference between mortality and the immortal neoplastic condition, with speculation that these may be tumor-suppressor genes and oncogenes. There is hope that identification of the genes will be revealing about processes involved in both carcinogenesis and clonal senescence (Norwood et al., 1990).

What does limited cell proliferation (clonal senescence) have to do with human life span? Tissues vary in their needs for cellular proliferation. Epithelial cells and blood cells are short lived and must be replaced constantly. Cells in other tissues, such as liver, proliferate intermittently (as in the repair of injury). The proliferation of cells in these cases is a part of somatic maintenance. Clonal senescence is an age-related decrement at the cellular level. Central nervous system neurons and heart muscle cells cannot proliferate after birth (Martin, 1977a).

The clonal senescence of fibroblasts, the cells in which it was first observed, has little to do with human mortality. Fibroblasts taken from nonagenarians are still able to divide about half as many times as fetal fibroblasts (Martin et al., 1970). It is recognized that wound healing is reduced in elderly people, but it is doubtful that this results from the clonal senescence of fibroblasts. Similarly, atrophy of skin and other epithelial surfaces and anemia (Lipschitz and Finch, 1985) are commonly seen in elderly people, but it is not likely that they result from clonal senescence.

Decline in the immune function with age that involves reduced cellular proliferation in response to stimulation may be related to clonal senescence, as observed in human T lymphocytes (Walford et al., 1981). Clonal senescence could have an effect on mortality through immune function.

## Age-related Functional Decrements at the Levels
## of Organs and Organisms

The idea of age-related functional decrements is already well established in this chapter. Such molecular and cellular processes, as the accumulation of unrepaired macromolecular damage, reduced immune function, reproductive senescence, and clonal senescence, have already been discussed. This section seeks to consider functional decrements at the level of organs, organ systems, and intact organisms. Such decrements have been reviewed extensively (Masoro, 1981; Shock, 1961), and the intention is not to repeat these reviews in a updated form but to provide a few examples to support some basic points.

Two problems are inherent in the investigation of function in aging. The first concerns functional decrements that occur because of diseases or consequent on diseases, in contrast to functional decrements that occur in the absence of disease—what have been described as functional decrements of normal aging (Shock, 1984). The extent of decrements found is inversely related to the rigor with which "normal" elderly subjects were selected. Thus, it is indicated in one widely cited paper (Brandfonbrenner et al., 1955) that the resting cardiac output (corrected for body surface area) falls 30 to 40 percent between the ages of 25 and 85, but it is stated in another paper (Rodeheffer et al., 1984) that it does not change significantly in healthy subjects. The latter study noted some more subtle age-related changes in cardiac function, such as a decrease in the maximum heart rate and an increase in end-systolic volume.

The second problem is that most studies on age and function are cross-sectional, examining some measurable indication of function in subjects presumed to be free of disease who are of different ages. The older subjects are survivors in that many of their cohort have already died, and they may have superior constitutions compared with those who have already died. It has been observed, for example, that the mean level of plasma cholesterol in men rises until about age 55, after which it begins to decline. Given what is known about hyperlipidemia as a risk factor in ischemic heart disease, it appears that those with the highest cholesterol levels die young, leaving a population with a lower mean cholesterol. The survivors of a cohort, the majority of which has died, do not describe the functional decrements that preceded death in those who did not survive.

These problems notwithstanding, age-related decrements in function have been described in virtually every system, as reviewed by Masoro (1981) and Shock (1961). There is, however, no common program of functional decline with age. In the absence of recognizable disease, the decrements appear and progress independently in each individual. The data, as with those of immune function, are characterized by much scatter. In any function studied, there are some subjects whose function overlaps measurements from much younger subjects, and there are many others with profound decrements compared with younger subjects. In view of the individual variability, these decrements cannot be considered as biomarkers of either aging or mortality (Baker and Sprott, 1988) in the sense that aging and mortality have the same course in all humans.

Some functional decrements are better tolerated than others. The failure to deliver oxygen because of cardiac, pulmonary, or vascular malfunction results rapidly in death. The failure to maintain the constancy of the ionic internal environment within a narrow range also results rapidly in death, with, for example, excitable membranes in the heart and brain functioning within a narrow range of intracellular and extracellular concentrations of sodium, potassium, and calcium, as well as pH (acidity).

Terminal organ failure affects homeostasis; however, earlier decrements of function reduce reserve capacity. In some cases the functional reserve is necessary for the expansion of voluntary effort and in the handling of stress. Thus, resting cardiac output can be expanded severalfold in healthy humans to maximum cardiac output as needed for exertion and as needed, for example, in the febrile state. When decrements in cardiac function reduce the maximum cardiac output to the resting cardiac output, the person can no longer get out of bed and cannot respond to any internal or external challenge that calls for increased cardiac output.

On the other hand, the two kidneys of the healthy younger adult have a three- to fivefold reserve capacity, but there is little need to expand renal function to maintain homeostasis in the face of voluntary exertion or external stress. Thus, the loss of one kidney far from exhausts the capacity to maintain homeostasis. Functional decrements in renal function with age have been described, although at each age a wide scatter in functional values for renal plasma flow and glomerular filtration rates is found (Lindeman, 1981). These functional decrements are usually not life threatening, and even specific renal diseases with terminal renal failure are not common causes of human death today.

To some extent the functional decrements are understandable in terms of age-related anatomical changes. Just as beef liver is tougher than calf liver, the collagen content of most tissues increases with age. This occurs because collagen replaces parenchymal cells and structures that die and are not regenerated, because of decreased collagen turnover, and because of increased collagen content with age of vascular structures and perivascular tissue. In the previous chapter, the formation of scars in organs consequent on specific diseases was discussed. Increased collagen deposition in the absence of specific disease is more diffuse and insidious. Variations on the themes of parenchymal depletion and vascular sclerosis are seen, with less functional tissue and with decreased nourishment of tissues being the consequences. These decrements do not lead to death in the 60s and 70s when heart disease, cancer, and cerebrovascular disease are the principal causes of death, but they may be more important in very elderly people, leading to death from the breakdown of homeostasis in the face of small challenges, stresses, and perturbations.

As with measurable functional decrements, there is no uniform schedule for these anatomical changes. In the study on the hearts of very elderly persons (over 90 years), cited in the previous chapter, Waller and Roberts (1983) found a great variety of changes, with a few very old hearts being indistinguishable from the hearts of much younger people.

In addition to the anatomical changes leading to decrements of tissue function, two other mechanisms have been suggested as contributing to functional decrements: reduced responsiveness of cells in older individuals and reduced signal transduction, by which cells fail to respond because they do not receive the necessary messages.

Considering intact organisms, function is often limited by the weakest system, or at least the weakest system on which integrated function depends. In the scattered values for more limited functions (e.g., organs and systems), some values from elderly people overlap the values found in the majority of much younger elderly people, as stated previously. The probability of any individual's retaining levels of function indistinguishable from much younger people in all important systems is small but finite. These are the people who can still run marathons and engage in other conspicuous feats. Even the strongest competitors in marathons in their 70s have records between three and four hours, compared with younger competitors who have records close to two hours (Fries and Crapo, 1981). There is much interest in the maintenance of high levels of integrated function to an advanced age for a larger percentage of the population. Terms, such as *healthy aging* (Schmidt, 1989) and *successful aging* (Rowe and Kahn, 1987), have been developed to describe the maintenance of a high level of integrated function to an advanced age.

Some longitudinal studies have been done to determine predictors, not only of longevity but also of the maintenance of a high level of integrated function (e.g., Shock, 1984; Busse and Maddox, 1985). In one such study (Guralnik and Kaplan, 1989) of midlife to elderly residents of Alameda County, California, the following were found to be predictors, not only of survival, but also of high levels of functioning 20 years later: race (not black), higher family income, absence of hypertension, absence of arthritis, absence of back pain, nonsmoking, normal weight, and the consumption of moderate amounts of alcohol (see Chapter 4).

## Conclusions

This chapter does not answer the question of what are the biomedical determinants of longevity. Genes and processes and biomarkers with strong genetic influences are all considered in their relationship to morbidity and mortality. Certainly much of mortality is influenced by alleles that affect the progress of life-threatening diseases. Much of survival is better considered "shortivity" (Editorial, *Lancet*, 1987) than longevity, even today.

A healthy genotype as defined by the absence of genes that predispose to the major fatal diseases is only relative. Mortality occurs later in these individuals, but it is not prevented. The DR1 histocompatibility allele in very old Okinawan Japanese, as described, may be an example of a healthy genotype because this allele precludes other alleles, some of which are involved in the pathogenesis of life-shortening diseases.

Age-related unrepaired and unreplaced wear and tear makes important contributions to mortality. Many processes are involved, and the progress of each process is so individually variable that a universal basis cannot be recognized presently. Somatic maintenance involves many functions, but in the balance somatic maintenance cannot keep pace with age-related damage and decrements. Age-related functional decrements are to be distinguished from functional decrements caused by diseases. Frailty contributes to mortality when challenges to homeostasis cannot be met. The challenges may come from major diseases of mortality, but as frailty progresses, fatal challenges may result from diseases or conditions that would not threaten a younger and less frail person. Are absolute limits to the human life span determined by wear and tear?

Within the biomedical limits of longevity of humans as individuals and as a species, other factors operate to determine the life span. These factors include behavior that may affect choices, and society that may provide formidable influences affecting behavior and may impose adverse conditions that are difficult to alter. Behavioral and societal factors affecting longevity are topics of the next chapter.

# 4

# Behavioral and Societal Determinants of Longevity

When a man lies dying, he does not die from the disease alone. He dies from his life.
CHARLES PÉGUY (1873–1914)
French poet and philosopher

Just as human longevity is affected by the biomedical factors discussed in the previous chapter, it is also affected by psychosocial factors. These are deeply rooted in human societies, as described by demographic data and in human behavior. They may shorten life spans by increasing the risks of mortality, or they may reduce the risks of mortality, thus permitting more of the potential maximum life span to be realized. In either case, behavioral and societal determinants of longevity act through the major causes of death, as described in Chapter 2.

Two approaches to psychosocial determinants of longevity will be taken here: (a) to examine behavioral contributions to the major causes of death, and (b) to examine groups that are more homogeneous than and different from the larger populations in aspects of longevity. Clues to determinants of life spans are seen from both approaches.

## The Major Causes of Death with Behavioral Determinants

The National Center for Health Statistics (Schoenborn and Cohen, 1986) identified several activities and conditions as "unhealthy habits" and "unhealthy practices." These are: smoking, alcohol consumption, sleeping less than six hours per day, never eating breakfast, daily snacking, a sedentary level of physical activity, and overweight. Of these, the first two can be most clearly associated with major causes of death. Much of the information offered about the causes of death is available in any textbook of medicine or pathology (e.g., Wilson et al., 1991; Cotran et al., 1989), but the latest data about vital statistics are included here.

*Diseases Associated with Cigarette Smoking*

The most recent estimate (1990) of the rate of cigarette smoking in the United States (Centers for Disease Control, 1992a) shows 25.5% of persons 18 and over—28.4% of men and 22.8% of women. The self-reported average number of cigarettes smoked per day by smokers was 19. It is estimated that another 4% of men and 1% of women use tobacco in other forms (Centers for Disease Control, 1989c). The number of former smokers is approximately equal to that of current smokers. Of people 18 and under in 1989 it is estimated that 11.8% of males and 11.2% of females had smoked within the preceding week (Centers for Disease Control, 1991b).

The rate of smoking has dropped rapidly. In 1983 it was estimated to be 32.3% (Schoenborn and Cohen, 1986). At that time it was estimated that 22.5% more of the population were former smokers and that 45.2% of people had never smoked. Of current smokers in 1983 it was estimated that 28.4% smoked fewer than 15 cigarettes per day, 44.8% smoked 15 to 24 cigarettes per day, 13.4% smoked 25 to 34 cigarettes per day, and 13.4% smoked 35 or more cigarettes per day. The prevalence of smoking was greater than 50% in the early 1960s. The prevalence of smoking varies widely among different groups in the United States population, and some of these differences will be discussed.

Cigarette smoke, with its nicotine, carcinogens, ciliotoxins, carbon monoxide, and particulates, is well recognized as an etiological agent or a risk factor in a variety of fatal diseases, the most prominent of which is lung cancer. Malignant tumors of the lung were listed as the cause of 125,522 deaths in the United States in 1986; an age-adjusted death rate from this cause of 54.1 per 100,000 of the population (National Center for Health Statistics, 1988). The association of lung cancer with smoking is well established, with the death rate from lung cancer being about 10-fold higher in men who have smoked one pack per day than in nonsmokers. There is a dose relationship: the death rate is 20 to 25 times higher in men who have smoked two or more packs per day, and the rate is related to the number of years of smoking. Although the highest rate of lung cancer mortality is in the 70- to 80-year-old group, in 1986 the greatest number of lung cancer deaths occurred in the 65- to 69-year-old group and nearly as many deaths occurred in the 60- to 64-year-old group (National Center for Health Statistics, 1988). Most people who will die of lung cancer are dead by the age of 70.

Most lung cancer is bronchogenic; it originates in the major branches of the bronchial tree. Several cell types are recognized, with differing associations with smoking history. Overall, it is estimated that about 85 percent of lung cancer is related to smoking. Higher incidences of cancer of the oral cavity, the esophagus, the kidney, the urinary bladder, and the pancreas are also found in smokers.

Smoking is a well-recognized risk factor in ischemic heart disease, with male smokers having a 70% increased risk of death from this cause. Smoking seems to interact synergistically with other risk factors in ischemic heart disease, which was listed as the cause of 520,750 deaths in 1986 (National Center for Health Statistics, 1988). Smoking is also a risk factor in cerebrovascular disease.

Chronic obstructive pulmonary disease includes a variety of conditions of the lungs, such as chronic bronchitis and emphysema—the enlargement of the air spaces at the expense of surface area for oxygen exchange. It was listed as the cause of 76,559 deaths in 1986 (National Center for Health Statistics, 1988), and it is estimated that 85% of cases of chronic obstructive pulmonary disease are associated with smoking.

It has also been observed that there is increased fetal loss by smoking mothers.

Overall the death rate of male smokers over the age of 35 is about 70% higher than that of male nonsmokers. The Centers for Disease Control has developed the concept of smoking attributable mortality. It includes all deaths from certain causes in smokers and former smokers. In 1988 (Centers for Disease Control, 1991c) it is estimated that 146,301 deaths of women and 285,319 deaths of men were smoking attributable, for a total of 434,175 deaths. This included an estimated 3,800 deaths from passive smoking. The smoking attributable deaths accounted for 20% of all mortality that year. 1.2 million years of life under age 65 were estimated to have been lost because of smoking attributable deaths. Smoking is a modifiable behavioral determinant of longevity. As successive cohorts age in which increasing numbers have stopped smoking and increasing percentages have never smoked, the mortality rates from smoking attributable causes can be expected to decrease, and life expectancy can be predicted to increase (see Chapter 7).

*Death Associated with the Consumption of Alcohol*

Most residents of the United States consume some alcohol. The National Center for Health Statistics (Schoenborn and Cohen, 1986), using criteria of the National Institute for Alcohol Abuse and Alcoholism, questioned persons 20 years and older in 1983 about their recent consumption of alcohol. They found that 33% consumed no more than one drink (defined as 0.5 ounce of ethanol) per month and were defined as abstainers. An additional 7% described themselves as former drinkers who drink no more, and the remaining 60% had consumed alcohol within the two weeks before questioning. The total alcohol consumed was divided by the time of the two-week period to give average daily rates of alcohol consumption. Those consuming 0.21 ounces per day or less of alcohol were defined as light drinkers and accounted for 29.5% of the total population. Those drinking 0.22 to 0.99 ounces per day were defined as moderate drinkers and accounted for 21.0% of the population. Heavy drinkers were those drinking more than 1.0 ounce per day of alcohol and accounted for 9.9% of the population. Of those defined as drinkers (light, moderate, and heavy), 37% drank five drinks or more in a single day at least once during the previous year, which was defined as a binge.

A genetic predisposition to alcoholism has long been suspected based on studies of families and of twins. An association has recently been reported between alcoholism and an allele of the gene for the human dopamine $D_2$ receptor. The rationale for looking at this gene was based on a role for neurotransmitters in alcohol-seeking behavior in experimental animals (Blum et al., 1990; Gordis et al., 1990). The finding remains controversial (Holden, 1991).

Ethanol, acetaldehyde, its principal metabolic product, and the congeners that are found in alcoholic beverages are toxic and depress function at every level from the cell to the intact organism. Alcohol abuse can be said to exacerbate any disease or pathological condition. In addition, nutritional deficiencies often co-exist with alcohol abuse.

The association of alcohol abuse with a major cause of death is apparent in liver disease. In 1986, there were 26,159 deaths attributed to chronic liver disease and cirrhosis (National Center for Health Statistics, 1988), placing this category among the 10 most common causes of death (see Table 2-2). It is a greater cause of death among young people than among elderly people. These deaths did not include 436 described as acute and subacute necrosis of the liver and 1,006 attributed to acute viral hepatitis. The category of chronic liver disease and cirrhosis included 921 deaths attributed to alcoholic fatty liver, 682 to acute alcoholic hepatitis, 7,409 to alcoholic cirrhosis, and 2,048 to alcoholic liver disease (unspecified). There were 12,746 deaths attributed to cirrhosis of the liver without mention of alcohol. Other causes of liver disease lead to hepatic failure, but there is evidence that alcoholic liver disease may be seriously under-reported. In a recent study from Oregon (Hopkins et al., 1989) death certificates showing chronic liver disease were questioned to determine previously unre-ported alcohol involvement. Alcoholic liver disease was originally listed in 56.9% of cases, but this increased to 82.4% as a result of questioning. Nationally 41.7% of death certificates of chronic liver disease mention alcohol, but one wonders what the death rate from chronic alcoholic liver disease actually is. The Oregon study yielded other revisions in causes of death as a result of queries by the state Office of Vital Statistics, but the increased implication of alcohol in liver disease was one of the most striking revisions.

Chronic abuse of alcohol is also associated with several disorders of the central nervous system and with cardiovascular diseases, including both arrhythmias when blood alcohol levels are high and a form of cardiomyopathy. It is associated with acute and chronic pancreatitis, but these conditions are not among the leading causes of death.

There is an association between alcohol drinking and accidental death and, as discussed, it constitutes the largest contribution to mortality in the United States.

A study described previously (see Chapter 3) suggested that mild consumption of alcohol was consistent with longer life and healthier aging (Guralnik and Kaplan, 1989), but this conclusion remains controversial (e.g., Lieber, 1984; Eichner, 1985; Colsher and Wallace, 1989). If there is an apparent beneficial effect from moderate alcohol consumption, it may be related to the higher income level of moderate drinkers and the fact that such people live longer and remain in better health (discussed later). It may also have to do with a role of moderate alcohol consumption in increasing the levels of high-density lipoproteins, which have a protective effect in ischemic heart disease.

*Other Unhealthy Practices*

The other unhealthy habits and practices listed play less certain roles in the major causes of death, although correlations between obesity and lack of exercise with heart disease have been described (e.g., Castelli, 1984). Some unhealthy habits are probably indicators of unhealthy life styles. For example, the National Center for Health Statistics (Schoenborn and Cohen, 1986) has shown that heavy smokers are more likely to get little sleep, skip breakfast, drink alcohol, and get little exercise. On the other hand, they are less likely to snack and be overweight.

*External Causes of Death: Accidents, Suicide, and Homicide*

Each of the external causes of death designated by the National Center for Health Statistics is one of the major causes of death in the contemporary United States. There are both societal and behavioral aspects of death from these causes, and there are large differences in their rates in defined groups in national populations.

ACCIDENTAL DEATH. Accidents accounted for 95,277 deaths in the United States in 1986 (National Center for Health Statistics, 1988), for a rate of 39.5 per 100,000. Accidental death is divided into transportation-related deaths (of which there were 50,925), or motor vehicle accident deaths (of which there were 47,865; rate 19.4/100.000), and other accidents (rate 19.7/100,000). Each of these categories ranks among the 10 most common causes of death.

The rate and number of motor vehicle fatalities has fallen since 1986 (Centers for Disease Control, 1992b), and the percentage of motor vehicle fatalities involving someone with a blood alcohol content of 0.01% or more has also fallen. In 1982, it is estimated that 57% of motor vehicle fatalities involved this level of blood alcohol, whereas in 1990, the percentage had declined to 50%. Still, it is estimated that 22,000 motor vehicle deaths were alcohol related, making this a more important cause of alcohol-related mortality than alcoholic chronic liver disease.

Other accidents, which accounted for about 44,000 deaths in 1986, included the following: falls, 14,444; poisoning, 5,740; fires, 4,835, suffocation, 3,692; "medical care misadventures," 2,873; and firearms, 1,432 (National Center for Health Statistics, 1988). Alcohol increases the risk of each of these (Nirenberg and Miller, 1984). The rate of both motor vehicle accident deaths and deaths from other accidents peaks in the 20- to 24-year-old age group and then increases again in elderly people.

SUICIDE. Suicide appeared on the death certificates of 30,904 individuals in 1986 (National Center for Health Statistics, 1988), with more than half of the cases involving firearms. The death rate from suicide reaches a plateau in the 20- to 24-year-old age group and remains quite constant through most of adult life. The ratio of men to women committing suicide is five to six. The highest rate of death from suicide is in men 80 to 84 years old and is about three times the rate in younger men. The suicide rate in blacks is lower than whites at all ages.

HOMICIDE AND LEGAL INTERVENTION. This category accounted for 21,731 deaths in 1986 (National Center for Health Statistics, 1988), of which 13,029 involved firearms. The homicide rate peaks in the 20- to 24-year-old age group and declines in older age groups.

## The Longevity of Smaller Populations

It is well recognized that the vital statistics of smaller populations, which are more homogeneous than national populations, can differ from those of the national populations. Sometimes the differences can be correlated with characteristics of the smaller populations. It must be recognized, however, that a correlation does not prove a causal relationship, and although many examples are presented, an effort is made not to overinterpret the correlations. Rather, questions raised by the correlations are pointed out.

### Sex/Gender

Since the first chapter of this book it has been apparent that men and women differ in their longevities in most populations. This is treated in detail in Chapter 5.

*Place of Residence: Political Subdivision*

National populations are defined geographically and politically and sometimes genetically. Large differences in longevity are found in different countries, with mean life expectancies at birth varying by a factor of more than two in the 1980s, and with life expectancies and socioeconomic development correlating (see Tables A-1 and A-2). There are large differences in the causes of death, as shown in Tables A-3 and A-4.

Within the United States, substantial differences in longevity are seen among the states of residence. Mean life expectancies at birth vary by a decade for men and by nearly seven years for women, with Hawaii followed by Minnesota being the most longevous states for both sexes and the District of Columbia having the shortest life expectancy for both sexes. The mean life expectancies at birth and at age 65 for each state are shown in Table A-5. The remaining years at age 65 vary for men by a little more than three years and for women by a little less than three years.

Interestingly, the states range by factors of two and more in age-adjusted mortality rates for major causes of death. Age-adjusted rates are used for these comparisons to avoid the effects of population age structure. As described in Chapter 2, all rates are adjusted to the age structure of the U.S. population in 1940. The use of age-adjusted rates permits the comparison of mortality rates from different times and from places with differing populations.

Table A-6 shows the mortality rates from several major causes in the different states and identifies those with the lowest and highest rates. There is some tendency for the rates from different causes to cancel each other out. For example, Delaware, which has a low death rate from strokes, has high male and female death rates from diabetes mellitus. An enigma is introduced by these findings because diabetes is a risk factor in cerebrovascular disease. Delaware also has a high death rate from breast cancer. Hawaii has the lowest male death rate from cardiovascular disease and the lowest female death rate from breast cancer, but the highest male and female death rates from stomach cancer. New Mexico has the lowest male and female death rates from homicide, but a high male death rate from suicide.

Why do the age-adjusted mortality rates from specific causes differ so much among the states? The variation seems surprising in view of the mobility of the population and some trends toward increasing uniformity of the population. There are, however, still differences in the characteristics of state populations.

The use of tobacco differs considerably from state to state, as shown in Table 4-1. The lowest prevalence of cigarette smoking, as determined by population surveys (Remington et al., 1989) in 1985, was 15% of people 20 and older in Utah. The next lowest prevalence, however, was 24% in Idaho and Nebraska.

**Table 4-1.  Variations in Tobacco and Alcohol Use by States**

| | Period of Study | Population | Range of Use | U.S. Average | States in Ascending Order (three of each) | |
|---|---|---|---|---|---|---|
| | | | | | Lowest Rates | Highest Rates |
| Prevalence of smoking | 1985 | Adults, 20+ | 15%–37% | 30.4% | UT, ID, NE | AK, KY, NV |
| Alcohol "Consumption" (see text) | 1985 | Persons 14+ | 1.53–5.34 gal/year | 2.65 gal/year | UT, WV, AR | NH, NV, DC |

*Sources*: Remington et al., 1989; Metropolitan Life, 1987f.

The highest prevalence was 37% in Nevada and 36% in Alaska and Kentucky. Wide variations are to be noted in the rates of smoking-attributable mortality in different states, with an enigma being provided by Alaska, which has a high prevalence of smoking but a low rate of smoking-attributable mortality (Centers for Disease Control, 1988). Alaska has one of the highest mortality rates from lung cancer, but it has a low mortality rate from cardiovascular disease, although smoking is recognized as a risk factor. In general, death rates from lung cancer correlate with the prevalence of smoking, whereas death rates from chronic obstructive pulmonary disease do not.

State per capita consumption of alcohol, calculated from the sales of alcoholic beverages divided by the state population aged 14 and over (Metropolitan Life, 1987f) is also shown in Table 4-1. The validity of the results is uncertain because it is not known how much of the alcohol purchased in a state was consumed in that state by residents of the state. It is well known that much liquor sold in states with low taxes on alcoholic beverages is carried out of state. The range, described as gallons of alcohol per person aged 14 and over in 1984, was from 5.34 in the District of Columbia to 1.54 in Utah. The national average was 2.65 gallons.

State differences in mortality rates cannot be explained by cigarette and tobacco consumption alone; they are more complex.

Similar differences occur within other countries. In a study of Western Europe (Van Poppel, 1981), male and female life expectancies were calculated for administrative units such as provinces, cantons, and *départements* in several countries, and substantial differences were found. Even more remarkable were sharp discontinuities that appeared at national borders, such as between Spain and Portugal, Sweden and Finland, and the Netherlands and West Germany. Shorter life expectancies were found in regions of cities with docks, of declining industries, and of concentrations of mines.

*Place of Residence: Urban/Rural*

Demographers have long recognized significant differences between urban and rural populations. Humans are becoming increasingly urbanized, although large national differences still exist as to the extent of urbanization. There are also national differences in the definition of urban populations, with residence in communities as small as 200 being defined as urban in some countries (United Nations, 1988). There is heterogeneity in the standards of living of both urban and rural residents. Substantial differences in longevity are seen within national populations according to urban and rural place of residence. Three patterns can be distinguished, as exemplified in Table 4-2. Because the published data (United Nations, 1988) were not age adjusted, the table provides age-specific mortality rates of people 65 to 69 years old for comparison of urban and rural residents. In a qualitative way similar urban and rural differences are seen in

**Table 4-2.  Examples of Mortality Rates, Urban and Rural Populations**

| Country and Year | Urbanization (%) | Population Studied | Mortality Rate of Population (per 100,000) | |
|---|---|---|---|---|
| | | | Urban | Rural |
| Similar Urban and Rural Mortality Rates | | | | |
| Austria, 1981 | 55.1 | Men, 65–69 | 34.5 | 35.2 |
| | | Women, 65–69 | 17.4 | 18.3 |
| France, 1982 | 73.4 | Men, 65–69 | 29.5 | 28.2 |
| | | Women, 65–69 | 12.5 | 12.1 |
| Greece, 1981 | 58.0 | Men, 65–69 | 30.5 | 29.0 |
| | | Women, 65–69 | 17.1 | 16.3 |
| Lower Urban Mortality Rates | | | | |
| Ireland, 1981 | | Men, 65–69 | 30.4 | 42.7 |
| | | Women, 65–69 | 17.9 | 24.3 |
| New Zealand, 1981 | 83.5 | Men, 65–69 | 27.1 | 73.6 |
| | | Women, 65–69 | 14.8 | 48.5 |
| Pakistan, 1976 | 28.1 (1980) | Men, 65–69 | 27.7 | 38.4 |
| | | Women, 65–69 | 22.5 | 19.6 |
| Republic of Korea, 1980 | 57.3 | Men, 65–69 | 54.7 | 63.5 |
| | | Women 65–69 | 23.1 | 29.3 |
| Lower Rural Mortality Rates | | | | |
| Mexico, 1979 | 66.3 (1980) | Men, 65–69 | 38.1 | 29.0 |
| | | Women, 65–69 | 26.1 | 23.4 |
| Paraguay, 1982 | 42.8 | Men, 65–69 | 28.0 | 11.0 |
| | | Women, 65–69 | 12.9 | 8.7 |
| Sri Lanka | 21.5 | Men, 65–69 | 63.4 | 21.4 |
| | | Women, 65–69 | 36.9 | 17.8 |

*Source*: United Nations, 1988.

death rates at other ages, including infant mortality. In the pattern usually seen in economically developed countries there are similar death rates for urban and rural people. Another pattern, however, shows a substantially lower death rate in the urban population, and yet another shows a substantially lower death rate in the rural population. One can speculate about differences in living conditions of the two populations with respect to poverty, hygiene, occupational hazards, crime, availability of health care, and the like as determinants of the patterns.

Urban and rural death rates are described as similar in the United States, but just as mortality rates differ among the states, there is a twofold variation in mortality rates within the limits of major cities. For example, Baltimore and Saint Louis have high death rates and Salt Lake City and San Jose have low death rates (National Center for Health Statistics, 1988). It must be recognized that the reported rates were not age adjusted, making their comparability questionable, but the age structures of the urban populations are not the sole determinants of the mortality rates in U.S. urban centers. There must be similar variations in death rates in rural populations.

*Race*

In 1987, the mean life expectancy at birth in the United States was 72.1 years for white men and 78.8 years for white women, compared with 65.4 years for black men and 73.8 years for black women—differences of 6.7 and 5.0 years, respectively. The white advantage in longevity persists up to old age (Metropolitan Life, 1989a). Several aspects of longevities of the two races are compared in Table 4-3.

Age-adjusted mortality rates for the major causes of death show large racial differences (Table 4-4). For most causes of death, the rates for whites are lower or much lower. There are racial differences in income, poverty, educational level, and unemployment, which can be taken as correlates of the longevity differences. There is a large racial difference in the prevalence of hypertension,

**Table 4-3.   Longevity Data, Blacks and Whites Compared**

|  | Black | | White | |
|---|---|---|---|---|
|  | Men | Women | Men | Women |
| Life expectancy at birth (years) (1987) | 65.4 | 73.8 | 72.1 | 78.8 |
| Mortality rate per 100,000 (1986) | 1,026 | 588 | 680 | 388 |
| Life expectancy at age 85 (years) (1987) | 5.7 | 7.0 | 5.1 | 6.3 |
| Mortality rate at age 85+ per 100,000 (1986) | 15,488 | 12,510 | 18,576 | 14,503 |

*Sources*: Metropolitan Life 1989a; National Center for Health Statistics, 1988.

**Table 4-4.   Mortality Rates from Common Causes, Blacks and Whites Compared**

| | Death Rate—Age Adjusted per 100,000 of Specified Population | | | | | | Ratio: Death Rates Both Sexes Black/White |
| | White | | | Black | | | |
| Cause | Both Sexes | Men | Women | Both Sexes | Men | Women | |
|---|---|---|---|---|---|---|---|
| Heart disease | 170.4 | 234.8 | 119.0 | 232.6 | 294.3 | 185.1 | 1.37 |
| Malignant neoplasms | 130.4 | 158.8 | 110.1 | 172.8 | 229.0 | 132.1 | 1.32 |
| Cerebrovascular dis-ease | 28.8 | 31.1 | 27.1 | 52.6 | 58.9 | 47.6 | 1.83 |
| Diabetes mellitus | 8.5 | 9.1 | 8.1 | 20.0 | 17.9 | 21.4 | 2.35 |
| Pneumonia and in-fluenza | 12.9 | 17.5 | 9.9 | 19.0 | 27.2 | 13.1 | 1.47 |
| Chronic obstructive pulmonary disease | 19.2 | 28.1 | 13.3 | 15.4 | 24.6 | 8.9 | 0.80 |
| Chronic liver disease and cirrhosis | 8.6 | 12.2 | 5.4 | 14.5 | 20.8 | 9.3 | 1.69 |
| Accidents | 34.5 | 51.1 | 18.4 | 42.1 | 66.9 | 21.0 | 1.22 |
| Suicide | 12.7 | 20.5 | 5.4 | 6.6 | 11.5 | 2.4 | 0.52 |
| Homicide and legal intervention | 5.6 | 8.4 | 2.9 | 32.3 | 55.9 | 11.8 | 5.77 |

*Source*: National Center for Health Statistics, 1988.

which is a risk factor in cardiovascular and cerebrovascular diseases (Metropolitan Life, 1989e). Infant mortality is higher in blacks (Metropolitan Life, 1988b). Smoking is more prevalent among black than white men, with 1990 figures being 32.6% and 27.9% respectively (Centers for Disease Control, 1992a), although it is a little lower among black women (21.2%) compared with white women (23.5%). The average self-reported cigarette consumption by black people of both sexes is lower. There is a residual excess mortality of black adults even after mortality rates are corrected for all recognized risk factors (Otten et al., 1990) and for family income (Sorlie et al., 1992).

A little-appreciated observation is that life expectancy is greater for very old (85+) blacks of both sexes than for very old whites, as shown in Table 4-3. In 1989, the life expectancy at age 85 was 5.1 years for white men, compared with 5.7 years for black men, and it was 6.3 more years for white women and 7.0 more years for black women. One can only guess about the reasons. Even for those born in 1990, the chances of reaching age 85 are about 60% for a black man and 70% for a black woman compared with whites (Metropolitan Life, 1992). Has some kind of selection for fitness left a healthier population of very old blacks? It can be shown that these very old blacks are still disadvantaged compared with their white contemporaries in terms of income (Rosenwaike,

1985). Alternatively, are errors made in reporting age so that very old blacks are not as old as claimed?

Racial differences in longevity are also seen between whites and other racial groups in Hawaii, which is the state with the greatest life expectancies and has some unusually low and unusually high mortality rates for some specific causes (see Table A-6). White, Japanese, Chinese, Filipino, and Hawaiian (Polynesian) people live there in close proximity, but as recognizable groups. There are large differences in the age-adjusted incidences of malignant neoplasms of various sites in these groups (Kolonel, 1988). Whites in Hawaii have twice the incidence of lung cancer as those of Japanese descent, although the prevalence of cigarette smoking is about the same in the two groups. Native Hawaiians have an even higher incidence of lung cancer than whites. Whites have approximately twice the incidence of breast (female) and prostatic (male) cancer as those of Japanese descent, but Japanese have more than twice the incidence of stomach cancer. The Oriental diet includes fermented and pickled foods, which may have a role in stomach carcinogenesis. In addition the high salt content of soy sauce and other Oriental foods may have a role in stomach cancer, as well as in hypertension (Weisburger, 1991).

A trend to a more white pattern of cancer incidence at various sites is seen when comparing Japanese in Japan, Hawaiian Issei, and Hawaiian Neisei, and diet is regarded as a major factor. Intakes of saturated fat and cholesterol correlate with the incidences of breast, prostatic, and lung cancer. Little genetic contribution can be detected.

A similar pattern is seen in heart disease (Yano et al., 1984), with the death rate from coronary heart disease in Hawaiian men of Japanese descent being about twice that of Japanese men in Japan but less than half that of whites living in the continental United States.

The racial composition of a population clearly affects the death rate and life expectancy in ways that defy simple explanation.

*Level of Income*

Demographers describe wealthier people as living longer. In a Canadian study (Millar, 1983), life expectancies and mortality rates were calculated for urban census tracts, using data from the 1970 Canadian census. All urban census tracts were divided into quintiles according to family income. Incomes in the highest quintile were above $11,500 and in the lowest quintile were below $7,400. Intermediate quintiles had family incomes between these values. Although the incomes appear to span less than a twofold range, the mean income in the highest quintile was above the figure defining the quintile, and the mean income in the lowest quintile was below the figure defining it. The range of incomes probably represents a range of living conditions from uncomfortable to reasonably comfortable.

The mean life expectancy at birth for men was 66.3 years in the poorest tracts and 72.5 years in the richest tracts, with expectancies in the intermediate tracts also correlating with family incomes. The annual age-adjusted male death rates differed by a factor of two, from 634 per 100,000 in the wealthiest tracts to 1,225 per 100,000 in the poorest tracts. Death rates were higher from all causes for men in the poorer tracts, including not only lung cancer, alcoholic liver disease, and violence, but also heart disease and cerebrovascular disease. As discussed in the next chapter, the income-related gradient in life expectancies and death rates was not as steep for women.

A recent study from the United States, based on the 1980 census, confirms the Canadian study (Sorlie et al., 1992). Mortality rate was found to be related to family income, and it was shown that the effect was prominent in the income range up to about 20,000 American dollars, beyond which the mortality rate changed very little with income. The relationship of income to mortality rate was most striking among younger people.

While the mechanisms leading to the correlations of mortality with income are complex, it should be noted that in the United States (Schoenborn and Cohen, 1986) the prevalence of smoking is highest at low income and education levels. Moderate alcohol use is the opposite.

## Marital Status

Demographers have recognized that married people live longer. In an extensive study of marital status and longevity in the United States, the National Center for Health Statistics (1970) found higher mortality rates for never married, divorced, separated, and widowed people at every age over 20 years, with rates up to 50 percent higher for the unmarried groups. Among white people, those who were divorced had the highest mortality rates, whereas among members of other races, those who were widowed had the highest mortality rates.

Since that study was published, married people have decreased from 71.7% of persons 18 and over (1970) to 61.4% (1990), with significant increases in the percent never married and the percent divorced. With the unmarried status becoming more common, the issue of marital status and longevity needs an up-to-date extensive study.

Another study (Foster et al., 1984) showed that men with substantially younger wives have longer life expectancies than men with older wives. One may wonder why such a correlation was seen, and it has been suggested that marriage selects for people in better health, especially marriage to a younger spouse. It has also been suggested that the marital state is more supportive of good health.

Another correlation is that 45.1% of men and 38.9% of women who are separated or divorced smoke cigarettes, compared with 28.7% of married men and 24.5% of married women (Centers for Disease Control, 1989c).

## Right and Left Handedness

It has been shown recently (Coren and Halpern, 1991) in a limited population of Americans that left-handed people had a remarkable eight-year shorter life expectancy than right-handed people. One can speculate as to whether this difference in life expectancies applies generally in developed societies and whether it reflects only the disadvantages of living in a largely right-handed world or whether it has additional bases.

## Life Styles

Life styles can include many things, and information about life styles is difficult to obtain for correlation with longevity data. Interesting studies of longevity and life style have been done by comparing members of two religious groups with the larger U.S. population. Both the Seventh-Day Adventist and the Mormon religions proscribe the use of tobacco and the consumption of alcoholic and caffeinated drinks. Members of these religious groups vary in their adherence to these and other teachings, but it seems safe to say that in the aggregate they differ from the larger U.S. population and that they are more homogeneous.

In addition to the above proscriptions, Mormons advise a strong family life, high educational achievement, and the limitation of sexual activity to the marital partner. Approximately 70% of the residents of Utah, which, as noted, has the lowest mortality rate from lung cancer and the lowest prevalence of smoking and per capita consumption of alcohol, is Mormon. It has been found that Mormons in Utah (Lyon et al., 1988) have 45% the incidence of what is described as cancer of smoking-related sites (mouth, pharynx, larynx, lung, esophagus, and urinary bladder) as does the entire U.S. population (smokers and nonsmokers). Non-Mormons in Utah have 92% the incidence of these tumors as the U.S. population. The incidence of cancer in some sites unrelated to smoking, such as breast and uterine cervix, is also lower in Mormons. In general, the death rates from nonsmoking-related cancer is 70% in Mormons, but the death rates from cancer of the prostate and lip and from malignant melanoma are higher among Mormons. There is a 65% mortality rate from ischemic heart disease in Mormons compared with all white people in the United States (Lyon et al., 1978).

In addition to the proscriptions on tobacco, alcohol, and caffeinated drinks, the Seventh-Day Adventist religion advises a diet that is largely vegetarian, with eggs and dairy products as the only acceptable sources of animal proteins. The mortality rates from cancer of the smoking-related sites among Seventh-Day Adventists are 30 to 40% the rates in the U.S. population, and the mortality rates for cancer of sites unrelated to smoking are 65 to 75% in Seventh-Day Adventists. The mortality rate from lung cancer is about 50% of the rate among non-smoking American who are not Seventh-Day Adventists, and an advantage is also observed in colorectal cancer (Phillips et al., 1980).

Among Seventh-Day Adventist men, the mortality rate from ischemic heart disease is 50 to 60% of the age-adjusted rate in the U.S. population. Little, if any advantage is seen, however, in the death rates from ischemic heart disease in Seventh-Day Adventist women (Fraser, 1988).

Surely, other groups—religious and otherwise—differ in life styles and mortality from national populations of which they are a part.

*Miscellaneous*

There have been many other studies seeking correlates of psychological and societal characteristics with longevity that have been reviewed (e.g., Cohen and Brody, 1981; Berkman, 1988) and are not considered comprehensively here.

An interesting example of these studies was carried out over a period of 25 years by Palmore and co-workers (1982) at Duke University. Two hundred fifty-two subjects, recruited in 1955 to 1959 in their 60s and 70s, admittedly not at random, were studied in detail initially and were then followed to determine their longevities. By 1982, most of the subjects had died, and it was attempted to correlate more than 50 initial findings with longevities as possible predictors of longevity. Many of the initial findings were related to health, leading to the obvious conclusion that those who were in better health upon entering the study lived longer. The strongest predictors for men were self-rated health (a stronger predictor than physician-related health), work satisfaction, and intelligence as measured by a standardized test. For women, the strongest predictors were health satisfaction, past enjoyment of sexual intercourse (!), and a rating of physical function determined by a physician. Other statistically significant correlations were observed for each sex; for example, finances and activity remote from the usual friends and family were of some predictive value in men and certain kinds of physical and social activities were predictive in women. The use of tobacco was a strong negative predictor of longevity in both sexes and strongly positive feelings about the importance of religion were a strong negative predictor in men, which appeared to be related to poorer health and lower socioeconomic standing. Some nonpredictors were mother's age at death (there was a weak correlation in men with father's age at death), obesity, marital status, and alcohol use.

This study must be valued for its longitudinal structure and the variety of variables observed, but it is of a small group of people, unrepresentative of any larger group. Some of the results, such as the nonpredictive value of marriage should probably be discounted in the face of the more extensive study described.

Another interesting study resulting in predictors of good health in later life was by Martin E.P. Seligman and co-workers at the University of Pennsylvania (Peterson et al., 1988). They had samples of writing by 268 Harvard students of the 1940s explaining some adverse event in their lives. The researchers analyzed what they called the explanatory style of 99 of the subjects on whom they could obtain current health data, using three pairs of extremes: stable (things have been and will always be bad) versus unstable; global (everything is bad) versus specific; and internal (things are bad because of me) versus external. Based on these criteria, styles were graded as pessimistic to optimistic, and a significant correlation was found between a pessimistic explanatory style in college and poor health beginning at about age 45. The correlation persisted up to the age of about 60, which was the age of the subjects shortly before the paper was written. No mention was made of a correlation between mortality and explanatory style. There is some speculation as to biomedical mechanisms that might underlie the correlation. There are many unanswered questions about the subjects and about the study, but the results are intriguing.

## Conclusions

As described in this chapter, psychological and societal factors have readily apparent effects on longevity. Sometimes individual choices are involved, including choices to avoid risks and choices for self-destructive behavior. Sometimes the choices of the individual are subject to strong societal influences, such as those imposed by race and socioeconomic level as well as by family and peers.

One wonders about roles for genetic factors in behavior and society, with some of the demographic data on longevity and on causes of death indicating genetic effects. The recent implication of a gene in alcoholism suggests a genetic component to individual choices involving some self-destructive behavior.

Some of the correlations described in this chapter between longevity and societal and behavioral factors operate through clear mechanisms, whereas the mechanisms are not obvious at all in others. Why should past sexual enjoyment be a correlate of female longevity? What is wrong with rural life in New Zealand? Why do mortality rates for common causes of death differ by factors of two and three in different states, with differences seen not only in comparing states as diverse as Hawaii and the District of Columbia, but also in states that would appear to differ very little? Such intriguing findings are no more than correlative, but it is tempting to think that they indicate something profound.

# 5

# Women Live Longer than Men

And now to all us women may Christ send
Submissive husbands, full of youth in bed,
And grace to outlive all the men we wed.

GEOFFREY CHAUCER (ca. 1340–1400)
Wife of Bath's Tale
*Canterbury Tales*

Casual observation of the population of developed countries gives the impression that women, in general, live longer than men. Most any assemblage of elderly people contains a larger proportion of women, and from the early pages of Chapter 1 extensive data have been provided to confirm this impression. Tables A-1 and A-2 show life expectancies for men and women at several ages from birth to 65 years in a variety of countries (United Nations, 1990), and in most cases life expectancies are greater for women, although there are some exceptions.

In the United States, life expectancies at birth in 1990 were 72.0 years for men and 78.8 years for women, with a longevity differential or a gender gap of 6.8 years (Metropolitan Life, 1992). The longevity differential, which is the topic of this chapter, has been reviewed recently from several points of view (Waldron, 1976, 1983; Lopez, 1983; Lopez and Ruzicka, 1983; Nathanson, 1984, 1990; Wingard, 1984; Hazzard, 1986, 1990; Metropolitan Life, 1988c; Smith and Warner, 1990).

## The Longevity Differential in Several Countries

The gender gap in longevity varies widely in national populations. In Table 5-1 the differences in female and male (female − male) life expectancies at birth in several national populations, as described in Tables A-1 and A-2, are shown. The list is in descending order of the differences.

**Table 5-1.  Differences in Female and Male Life Expectancies at Birth in Countries Shown in Tables A-1 and A-2**

| Country | Year of Data | Life Expectancy at Birth (years) | | Difference (female–male) |
|---|---|---|---|---|
| | | Male | Female | |
| Former USSR | 1984–1985 | 62.9 | 72.7 | 9.8 |
| Finland | 1985 | 70.1 | 78.5 | 8.4 |
| France | 1983–1985 | 71.0 | 79.2 | 8.2 |
| Czechoslovakia | 1984 | 67.1 | 74.3 | 7.2 |
| Botswana | 1981 | 52.3 | 59.7 | 7.4 |
| Canada | 1980–1982 | 71.9 | 79.0 | 7.1 |
| United States | 1988 | 71.4 | 78.3 | 6.9 |
| Austria | 1985 | 70.4 | 77.3 | 6.9 |
| Italy | 1981 | 71.0 | 77.8 | 6.8 |
| Netherlands | 1984–1985 | 72.8 | 79.5 | 6.7 |
| Iceland | 1983–1984 | 74.0 | 80.2 | 6.2 |
| United Kingdom | 1983–1985 | 71.8 | 77.9 | 6.1 |
| Denmark | 1984–1985 | 71.6 | 77.5 | 5.9 |
| Sweden | 1982 | 73.8 | 79.7 | 5.9 |
| Japan | 1985 | 74.8 | 80.4 | 5.6 |
| Guatamala | 1975–1979 | 55.1 | 59.4 | 4.3 |
| Greece | 1980 | 72.1 | 76.3 | 4.2 |
| Israel | 1984 | 73.1 | 76.6 | 3.5 |
| Malawi | 1977 | 38.1 | 41.2 | 3.2 |
| Sierra Leone | 1980–1985 | 32.5 | 35.5 | 3.0 |
| Mali | 1976 | 46.9 | 49.7 | 2.8 |
| Ecuador | 1974–1979 | 59.5 | 61.8 | 2.3 |
| Algeria | 1983 | 61.6 | 63.2 | 1.6 |
| Syria | 1976–1979 | 63.8 | 64.7 | 0.9 |
| Pakistan | 1976–1978 | 59.0 | 59.2 | 0.2 |
| Bangladesh | 1984 | 54.9 | 54.7 | −0.2 |
| India | 1976–1980 | 52.5 | 52.1 | −0.4 |
| Iran | 1976 | 55.8 | 55.0 | −0.8 |
| Nepal | 1981 | 50.9 | 48.1 | −2.8 |

*Source*: United Nations, 1988.

In developed countries the longevity differences vary over a twofold range from about 5 to 10 years. The gap is greatest in the former Soviet Union where men have shorter lives than in other developed countries, and where women do not have very long lives either. The third country from the top of the list, however, is France where women have unusually long lives. The longevity differential is small in Greece, where men have relatively long lives. In Japan, the most longevous national population of all, the gap is small, with both men and women having greater life expectancies at birth than any other national population. Both male and female longevities must be considered in examining national differences in gender gaps. Neither a small nor a large gap by itself reveals much about longevity or suggests much about the quality of life.

Women also have greater life expectancies in most of the less-developed countries. Life expectancies are shorter for both sexes, but commonly the gender gap is about the same 5 to 10 percent of the life expectancy at birth, as seen in developed countries. There are a few countries, however, in which the ratio of female to male life expectancies is close to unity or in which the male life expectancy is actually greater than the female life expectancy, as shown at the bottom of Table 5-1.

*Countries with Shorter Female Longevity*

Because most of this chapter is about why women live longer than men, it is worth pausing at this point to consider the few national populations in which the reverse is the case. The United Nations publication, *The State of World Population 1989* (Sadik, 1989) focuses on women and provides an appalling description of the treatment of girls and women in some countries where the gender gap is small or reversed and in some other less developed countries.

Of the poor countries with high childhood death rates shown in Table 5-2, some have similar rates for boys and girls, whereas in others the rates for girls are up to 50% higher. In Bangladesh boys under five years of age are given 16% more food than girls, and there is evidence that this difference increases in times

**Table 5-2.  Sex Differences in Child Mortality:**
**Countries with High Child Mortality**

| | Mortality Rates (per 1,000 in age group) of Children Aged | | | | | |
| | 1–2 Years | | | 2–5 Years | | |
| Country | Female | Male | Ratio Female–Male Rates | Female | Male | Ratio Female–Male Rates |
|---|---|---|---|---|---|---|
| Pakistan | 40.4 | 26.1 | 1.55 | 54.4 | 36.9 | 1.47 |
| Haiti | 27.6 | 30.6 | 0.90 | 61.2 | 47.8 | 1.26 |
| Bangladesh | 35.4 | 26.0 | 1.36 | 68.6 | 57.7 | 1.19 |
| Nepal | 55.0 | 49.2 | 1.12 | 60.7 | 57.7 | 1.05 |
| Peru | 33.4 | 33.4 | 1.00 | 30.8 | 28.8 | 1.07 |
| Turkey | 34.2 | 21.2 | 1.61 | 19.5 | 18.4 | 1.06 |
| Senegal | 77.3 | 76.5 | 1.01 | 106.8 | 107.0 | 1.00 |
| N. Sudan | 28.2 | 32.9 | 0.86 | 35.7 | 36.4 | 0.98 |
| Lesotho | 24.4 | 35.3 | 0.69 | 26.6 | 29.3 | 0.91 |
| Indonesia | 28.2 | 32.3 | 0.87 | 40.1 | 52.6 | 0.76 |

*Source*: Sadik, 1989.

of famine. In India, girls are more than four times as likely as boys to be suffering from malnutrition, but only about 2% as likely to be taken to a hospital. In developing countries as a whole, 65% of girls of appropriate age are in primary schools compared with 78% of boys, and 37% of girls of appropriate age attend secondary schools compared with 48% of boys. In Pakistan and the Yemen Arab Republic there are more than three times as many boys as girls in secondary school. Parents with limited resources invest more in their sons than their daughters, presumably because of expectations of later support.

The child-bearing years as well as infancy and childhood are times of high female mortality in less-developed countries. The maternal mortality rate in Africa is nearly 100 times the maternal mortality rate in North America (per 1,000 live births), and given that the fertility rate in Africa is more than three times higher than in North America, the lifetime risk of maternal death in Africa is 300 times greater.

In many of the less-developed countries, even survival past childhood and the child-bearing years does not provide much female longevity advantage. The life expectancy at age 65, which is about four years longer for women compared with men in most developed countries, is miniscule in most but not all of the countries that have negligible or reversed gender gaps in life expectancy at birth (see Table A-2).

The United Nations study (Sadik, 1989) indicates that self-determination by women has a major role in reducing female mortality. Education, family planning with at least a four-year spacing of pregnancies, the avoidance of early pregnancy, medical care, and nutrition correlate with lower maternal and lower infant mortality. Declining fertility rates and birth rates are correlated with increased female longevity, but the report states that fertility rates remain high or are actually increasing in countries such as Nepal, Pakistan, Afghanistan, Malawi, and other countries of subsaharan Africa and West Asia. Evidence (Food and Agriculture Organization, 1992) that undernutrition is decreasing in most of the developing countries (except Africa) suggests that some of the basis for shorter female longevity in these countries is changing. From these studies it must be concluded that, if given half a chance, women will live longer than men.

## The Gender Gap in the United States Since the Nineteenth Century

The magnitude of the gender gap in longevity is a recent phenomenon, but the life expectancy of women was greater than men in Massachusetts in 1850. Life expectancies at birth were then 38.5 years for men and 40.5 years for women (Bureau of the Census, 1975). As it is today in some less-developed countries (see Table A-2), the mean life expectancy of a member of either sex reaching the age of 20 years was 40 additional years. During the second half of the nineteenth century life expectancy at birth in Massachusetts for each sex increased eight or nine years to 46.1 years for men and 49.4 years for women in 1900, with a gender gap of 3.3 years.

Figure 5-1 describes the gender gap in life expectancies at birth in the United States from 1900 to the present. In 1900 it was 2.0 years in the reporting states (see Chapter 1), with life expectancies at birth being 46.3 years for men and 48.3 years for women. The gender gap decreased to 1.0 year in 1920, related to greater female mortality during the influenza epidemic. It then climbed steadily to 7.8 years in 1975, but since that year it has fallen to 6.8 years in 1989 and 1990 and as estimated for 1991 (Metropolitan Life, 1988a, 1990, 1992).

Women more than men have benefited from the improvements in living standards, public health, and medical care that have occurred in this century and that changed mortality so much, as discussed in Chapters 1 and 2.

## Details of the Longevity Differential
## in the Contemporary United States

So far in this chapter, life expectancies have been used to describe the gender gap in longevities, but other kinds of data also provide evidence of a significant longevity differential.

### Mortality Rates

Approximately (not exactly) equal numbers of boys and girls are born, and everyone dies, therefore, the number of deaths of men and women in the United States is approximately equal in a given year (1,104,005 men and 1,001,356 women in 1986), but women are older when they die. Death rates were 941 men and 809 women per 100,000, for a ratio of 1.16. Because women live longer than men, however, age-adjusted rates were 709 men and 407 women per 100,000, for a ratio of 1.74 (National Center for Health Statistics, 1988).

American women have lower mortality rates than men at every age, but the ratio of male to female rates varies strikingly at different ages, as shown in Figure 5-2. The mortality rate for men is about three times that of women in the adolescent–young adult (15 to 24 years) age group, whereas the male rate is less than 1.3 times the female rate in people over the age of 85. This suggests that whatever factors are involved in the gender gap have largely finished operating in the very old. Patterns similar to that shown in Figure 5-2 for the United States, with a large peak in the mortality rate ratio in young adult life and a second smaller peak in the ratio in early elderly life are also seen in Canada, Australia,

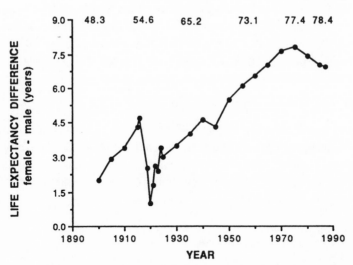

**Figure 5-1.** Changes in the gender gap in longevities during the twentieth century. Differences in life expectancies of women and men (female–male) in the United States are shown. The numbers at the top show life expectancies for women at birth at 20-year intervals since 1900 and for 1987. (Source: National Center for Health Statistics, 1990.)

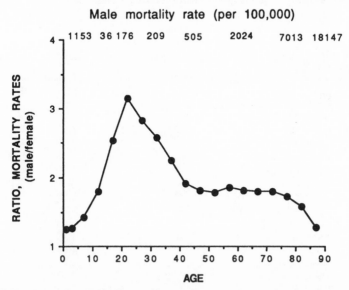

**Figure 5-2.** Ratio of mortality rates with age. The ratios (male–female) of age-adjusted mortality rates at different ages are shown. The ratio is greater than 1.0 at every age but varies widely. At the top are shown age-specific male mortality rates at several ages. (Source: National Center for Health Statistics, 1988.)

Denmark, and some other developed countries. In the United Kingdom, Belgium, and the Netherlands the excess male mortality in young adult life is not so great. In countries of Eastern Europe the high male mortality of early adult life falls off gradually, with the ratio in the elderly years forming a shoulder on the young adult peak rather than a distinct peak (Lopez, 1983; Wingard, 1984).

*Sex Differences in Mortality from Specific Causes*

Men have greater age-adjusted death rates from each of the 10 major causes of death in contemporary United States, as shown in Table 5-3. The ratio of male to female rates, however, varies from near unity from deaths attributed to diabetes mellitus and strokes to 2.07 for cardiovascular disease to 3 and more for deaths due to lung cancer, homicide, and suicide.

*A Gender Gap in Prenatal Mortality*

The sex ratio (male to female) at conception has been variously estimated to be between 1.15 and as high as 2.0. The reasons for this male preponderance are obscure and cannot be explained by a greater abundance of sperm containing the

**Table 5-3.  Sex Differences in Mortality Rates:**
**Major Causes of Death**

| Cause of Death | Mortality Rates (per 100,000) Age Adjusted, 1986 | | Ratio of Mortality Rates |
|---|---|---|---|
| | Men | Women | Male–Female |
| Ischemic heart disease | 166.9 | 80.7 | 2.07 |
| All cancer | 163.6 | 111.4 | 1.47 |
| Lung cancer | 59.8 | 22.9 | 2.61 |
| All other cancer | 103.8 | 88.5 | 1.17 |
| Cerebrovascular disease | 33.5 | 29.0 | 1.15 |
| Accidents | 52.5 | 18.7 | 2.81 |
| Motor vehicle accidents | 28.5 | 10.6 | 2.69 |
| Chronic obstructive pulmonary disease | 27.6 | 32.8 | 2.16 |
| Pneumonia and influenza | 18.4 | 10.3 | 1.79 |
| Diabetes mellitus | 9.9 | 9.3 | 1.06 |
| Suicide | 19.3 | 5.1 | 3.78 |
| Chronic liver disease | 13.0 | 5.9 | 2.20 |
| Homicide | 12.9 | 4.1 | 3.39 |
| All causes | 709 | 407 | 1.74 |

*Source of mortality rates*: National Center for Health Statistics, 1988.

Y chromosome or greater success of these sperm in penetrating ova (Neel, 1990). The ratio in spontaneous abortuses is about 1.3 male per female fetus, whereas the sex ratio at birth is about 1.05, indicating a substantial excess of male mortality in utero (McMillen, 1979; Hassold et al., 1983).

The causes of this early male die-off are unknown. Considering the chromosomes of abortuses, Hassold and colleagues (1983) found a 1.3-fold male excess among those that were chromosomally normal but a smaller male preponderance among those with a variety of autosomal trisomys. Neel (1990) doubts that hemizygosity (elaborated later) for the X chromosome in males and lethal recessive X-linked genes for diseases could explain the excess male die-off.

*Sex Ratios at Different Ages*

The sex ratio of 1.05 males per female at birth decreases through life, predictably, as a result of the greater male mortality rate at every age, as shown in Figure 5-3 (Bureau of the Census, 1987). Few deaths occur in the early years of life, and it is not until the age of 30 that the sex ratio reaches unity. Even at age 65 it is still 0.8 men per woman. During the ages 65 to 85, however, when most deaths occur, the ratio changes rapidly, therefore, in the over 85-year-old age group there are more than two women per man. There are nearly three women per surviving man as age 100 is approached.

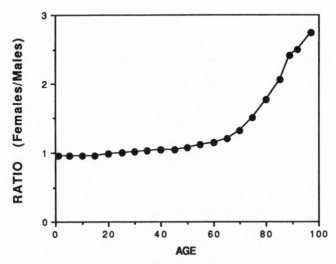

**Figure 5-3.** Sex ratio in the United States with age. The ratio of women to men in the population according to 1980 census results at different ages is shown. (Source: Bureau of the Census, 1987.)

## Sex and Human Development

What are the basic differences in men and women? In the next section it is considered how development results in the differences and how they could contribute to the gender gap.

### Chromosomal (Karyotypic) Sex

Mammalian sex is determined chromosomally at the moment of conception, whereas in some lower animals sex has environmental determinants (Bull, 1983). Each human cell contains 46 chromosomes, of which 44 (22 pairs) are similar in men and women, and are called autosomes. The remaining two are called sex chromosomes, and their complement is different in men and women. Each female cell contains two X chromosomes, one derived from the ovum of the mother and one from the sperm of the father. The production of ova, the female gametes, results in a halving of the chromosome number (meiosis) to one set of autosomes and one X chromosome, which may be of maternal or paternal origin (haploidy). Each male cell contains one X chromosome that is derived from the mother and a Y chromosome that comes from the father's sperm. Sperm contain one set of autosomes and either an X or a Y chromosome. A female child results from the fertilization of an ovum by a sperm containing an X chromosome, and a male child results from the fertilization of an ovum by a sperm containing a Y chromosome.

The chromosomal content of the fertilized egg sets in motion a cascade of events, as shown diagrammatically in Figure 5-4, that continues through life and results in a male or a female individual. What are the genes on the X and Y chromosomes that act to determine sex? The X chromosome is about three times the size of the Y chromosome, and most of its complement of genes has nothing to do with femaleness (Sandberg, 1983). It has genes for vital functions that occur in every cell such as enzymes in the metabolism of carbohydrates, amino acids, and nucleotides. It also has genes for specialized functions of differentiated cells such as the synthesis of blood clotting factor VIII by the liver and dystrophin in skeletal muscle cells. Although each cell of a mammalian female contains two X chromosomes, most of the genes on one X chromosome in each cell are inactivated early (100 to 1,000-cell stage) in development (Lyon, 1972; Gartler and Riggs, 1983). Usually inactivation is a random process in eutherian mammals, and the pattern of inactivation in each cell is passed on to its daughter cells (Holliday, 1987a), leaving the female mammal a mosaic of functionally hemizygous cells, some of which express the genes of the maternal X chromosome and some the genes of the paternal X chromosome.

The Y chromosome has few genes that are expressed (Sandberg, 1985). Much

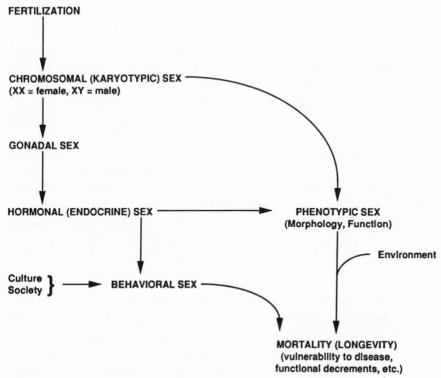

**Figure 5-4.** Cascade of critical developmental events leading to human males and females. This diagram illustrates the development of the sexes as described in the text.

of its DNA is heterochromatic and composed of repeated base sequences. There is sufficient homology of its base sequences with the X chromosome that the short arms of the two chromosome pair in meiosis. The mammalian male is hemizygous for the genes of its single X chromosome, having only a single allele for each X-linked gene. The Y chromosome is essential for male development, and it has long been recognized that deletions in the juxtacentromeric portion of the short arm of the Y chromosome are associated with the failure of testicular development. Recently, a specific gene in this location has been identified as involved in testicular differentiation (Burgoyne, 1989; Koopman et al., 1989; Palmer et al., 1989). There appear to be nearby genes for spermatogenesis and for stature (Sandberg, 1985). In the absence of this part of the Y chromosome what is called a *streak gonad* develops. Although it is not correct to say that any mammal without a Y chromosome is a female, the specific contributions of two X chromosome to ovarian development and other aspects of femaleness are not well defined (Sandberg, 1983; Federman, 1987).

*Gonadal and Hormonal Sex*

Testicular development with the ability to produce the principal androgenic male steroid hormone, testosterone, is essential for further features of male development (Fig. 5-4). The female steroid sex hormones, the estrogenic and progesteroid hormones, are produced by the ovaries and are needed for female development. In the case of each sex, gonadal function requires neuroendocrine stimulation, and the hormonal changes through the life span are based on both primary changes in the gonads and changes in the neuroendocrine regulation of gonadal function. As described previously (see Chapter 3), the supply of germ cells of women is exhausted at the time of reproductive senescence, and in their absence, ovarian hormones are not formed. In men the depletion of the germ cells (precursors of sperm) is more gradual, and the production of androgenic hormones is not dependent on sperm production, therefore, the formation of testosterone can continue to a more advanced age (Finch, 1987).

*Phenotypic Sex*

There are organs directly dependent on sex hormone secretion for development and maintenance including the uterus, breasts, and penis, and sex hormones also affect hair patterns, muscle development, and bone growth and mineralization. They modulate immune responses and the handling of cholesterol (discussed later). Their influences change through the life span depending on secretory levels and on responsiveness of target tissues.

*Behavioral and Societal Sex*

Sex hormones have major effects on behavior. This is seen in lower animals in which there are widespread behavioral differences between the sexes in territoriality, aggressiveness, socialization, vocalization, choice of mating partner, mating behavior, and the raising of young. Sex hormones affect the central nervous system both prenatally and postnatally (Ehrhardt and Meyer-Bahlberg, 1981; Maclusky and Naftolin, 1981), and in humans sex hormones also have large effects on behavior (Rubin et al., 1981).

Family, culture, and society influence human gender-related behavior, with role models, education, expectations, and lifetime experience interacting with the behavioral effects of sex hormones.

## Why do Women Live Longer than Men?

There are large recognizable contributions to the gender gap in longevity that derive from the cascade of sexual development as described and shown in Figure 5-4.

## Cardiovascular Diseases and the Handling of Cholesterol

The age-adjusted death rates from ischemic heart disease differ by a factor of two in men and women, as shown in Table 5-3. As discussed in Chapter 2 (see Fig. 2-1), the mortality rate from ischemic heart disease increases exponentially with age. Although this is the case for both sexes, and although ischemic heart disease is the most common cause of death of both sexes, the age-related rate increase in women lags behind that in men by 5 to 10 years in the United States. The rate in women catches up with that in men at an advanced age, but at younger ages when most deaths occur, this lag makes a large contribution to the gender gap, as is shown in Figure 5-5.

There is a biological basis for the male to female differences in ischemic heart disease mortality that is related to the modulation of cholesterol handling by sex hormones. As described previously (see Chapter 2), hyperlipidemia and hyper-cholesterolemia are risk factors in ischemic heart disease, presumably acting through atherogenesis that affects the aorta and its major branches including the coronary arteries. Evidence for the effects of sex hormones on ischemic heart disease is largely correlative, but it is persuasive (Hazzard, 1986, 1990).

The range of serum cholesterol values falling within the 5th to the 95th percentiles is slightly lower in premenopausal women than men of comparable age (range for women at age 39: 141 to 245 mg/dL; for men: 146 to 270 mg/dL) (Wilson et al., 1991). The values for the low-density lipoprotein (LDL) choles-

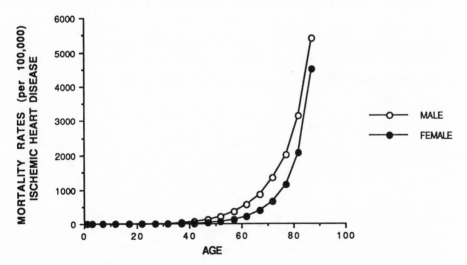

**Figure 5-5.** Male and female mortality rates from ischemic heart diseases with age. Based on age-specific mortality rates from ischemic heart disease of the United States population in 1986, the difference between age-related mortality of men and women is shown. The mortality rate increases with age more slowly in women. (Source: National Center for Health Statistics, 1988.)

terol, which correlate with the incidence of ischemic heart disease (see Chapter 2), are 75 to 172 mg cholesterol/dL for women and 81 to 189 mg cholesterol/dL for men. After menopause the female values rise to the male range. The serum high-density lipoprotein (HDL) cholesterol values, which correlate negatively with the incidence of ischemic heart disease, are higher in women than in men throughout life.

Effects of sex hormones on cholesterol handling, as suggested by these levels and by the increase in female LDL levels at the menopause, are also indicated by lipoprotein changes in cases in which hormonal treatments are administered for medical reasons. Elderly women are sometimes treated with anabolic steroids for osteoperosis and muscle atrophy, and increases are seen in LDLs and decreases in HDLs. Postmenopausal women taking conjugated estrogens have lower LDL and higher HDL levels than women not taking them. A study showed mortality from cardiovascular disease in a group treated with estrogens to be 33% that of an untreated group, and another study found it to be 43% (Hazzard, 1986, 1990).

Old men with prostatic cancer are sometimes treated with estrogenic hormones to inhibit tumor growth, and there is a fall in LDL levels. Estrogen therapy has its risks, however, in the form of increased blood clotting, especially in treated men.

## Society and Behavior

A discussion of societal and behavioral contributions to the gender gap shares some similarities and problems with the discussion in Chapter 4 of psychosocial determinants of longevity. There are real male to female differences in mortality rates from specific causes that have societal and behavioral components. These include the so-called external causes of death—accidents, homicide, and suicide—in which age-adjusted male mortality rates are three and more times female rates. Most mortality in the adolescent and young adult age groups results from these causes. The rate from suicide by men aged 80 to 84 is nearly 10 times the rate by women of the same age.

Then there are smoking and alcohol abuse, with higher male rates and predictably higher male death rates from lung cancer and chronic liver disease. The opinion has been expressed (Holden, 1983; Waldron, 1986) that male and female smoking differences are a major contribution to the gender gap.

Behavioral and societal contributions to the gender gap are associated with greater risk-taking and self-destructive behavior by men and possibly greater self-protective behavior by women. Smoking and alcohol abuse are obvious self-destructive acts in which men exceed women. Men wear seat belts (Williams and Lund, 1986) and seek medical and dental attention less often than women (Verbrugge, 1983; Verbrugge and Wingard, 1987). Men engage in more dangerous occupations. Of the approximately 7,000 occupational fatalities in the United

States between 1980 and 1985, 94 percent were men (Bell et al., 1990). Ninety-five percent of the prison population in the United States is male (Bureau of the Census, 1989), and in wartime, men have borne virtually all of the battlefield casualties through history.

What is it about maleness that has resulted in these differences? The question will not be pursued here except to note that, in general, greater male size and strength are consequences of the cascade of sexual development, with likely determinants that are both chromosomal and hormonal. Do the sex-related behavioral differences that are so obvious in animals, have counterparts in human male behavior?

There are more homogeneous groups within national populations with different gender gaps. The gender gap among blacks is now larger than among whites in the United States (Metropolitan Life, 1989a). The gender gap is negligible among Seventh-Day Adventists who, as described in Chapter 4, have proscriptions as to the use of tobacco and the intake of alcohol and meat, and who live longer than the American population (Phillips et al., 1980; Berkel and deWaard, 1983; Fraser, 1988).

The Canadian study of Millar (1983), described in Chapter 4 as relating income and longevity, shows a greater gender gap at lower income levels. At the lowest income level studied, the gender gap was 8.3 years, whereas at the highest level the gender gap was 5.0 years. The ratio of the male age-adjusted death rate to the female death rate was 2.26 in the lowest income group and 1.77 in the highest income group, indicating that income differences have a greater effect on male than on female longevity. This finding was confirmed in the recent study from the United States cited in Chapter 4 (Sorlie et al., 1992). There is an obvious contribution from smoking (Schoenborn and Cohen, 1986) through lung cancer, where the rate is higher in low income groups and where the income effect is more pronounced among men. There is also a substantial contribution in mortality rates from external causes, and there are differences in mortality rates from ischemic heart disease and cerebrovascular disease.

It has been stated (Nathanson, 1990) that a large part of the gender gap in the United States is the contribution of blue collar men, who constitute higher risks in several aspects of longevity.

There is current interest in whether the changing roles of men and women in Western societies may alter societal and behavioral contributions to the gender gap. A focus has been the possible stress of female work force participation, especially as it has been added to more traditional female roles of parenting and care giving. The literature on the subject (e.g., Verbrugge and Madans, 1985; Passannante and Nathanson, 1987; Waldron and Jacobs, 1988, and their references) suggests that work force participation is consistent with better female health, although exceptions have been noted. There are uncontrolled factors operating in these studies such as financial well-being and social class, and work force participation selects for people in better health.

There is a paucity of studies on stress in which gender is a variable. Stress can operate through adrenal cortical hormone secretion to reduce immune function in body defenses against infectious organisms and possibly against tumors and also to moderate harmful immune reactions. There have been studies correlating a sense of control with longevity and with stronger immune function (Rodin, 1986), but these have not addressed the mechanisms behind the correlations. It is not known if there are gender differences in the perception of stress, the mechanisms to cope with it, and the somatic consequences of stress. The studies have not been done, and given the complexity of the issues and the problems of doing research of this kind, the answers will be slow in coming.

*Some Male to Female Differences Making Uncertain but Possibly Significant Contributions to the Gender Gap*

THE IMMUNE SYSTEM. Aside from the speculation on gender differences in immune function in response to stress, there are other sex-based differences in immune function that change with age and could contribute to the gender gap.

Some (reviewed by Weksler, 1990) state that several aspects of the immune function are stronger in women than in men. These include both cellular responses, such as skin graft rejection and T-lymphocyte proliferation in response to mitogens, and humoral responses such as specific antibody synthesis. Although these phenomena could offer potential advantages to female longevity, it must be recognized that aberrant immune responses associated with autoimmunity are more common both in female mice and in women (Talal, 1981). Sex hormones play important roles in sex-related immune differences, with estrogens increasing immune responses but also accelerating the progress of autoimmune diseases. Castration and treatment with male hormones retard autoimmune diseases in female mice.

In humans there is some evidence that immune functions are less affected by age in women than in men. A study of T-lymphocyte subsets shows less decline in cell numbers with age in women (Mascart-Lemone et al., 1982).

There may be a genetic as well as a hormonal basis for a more robust immune function in women. Several genes important in both T- and B-lymphocyte function have been mapped to the X chromosome (Buckley, 1986; Waldman, 1986). The functions of these genes are best recognized from the hereditary immunodeficiencies that occur when there are mutant alleles. The most commonly occurring is Bruton's agammaglobulinemia, which is a fatal disease in early life in boys because of the single X chromosome. It is not a significant problem for heterozygous girls who have two X chromosomes. They are phenotypic mosaics

with respect to X chromosome expression (see above), but in the female heterozygote there is cell selection that occurs during B-lymphocyte proliferation so
that the B lymphocytes expressing the allele with the intact gene populate the
heterozygote to the virtual exclusion of B lymphocytes expressing the mutant
allele (Fearon et al., 1987).

In the next section another mechanism is discussed by which the female
karyotype may increase late life cellular proliferative potential in women. This
could increase immune function, which includes cell proliferation.

DOES CHROMOSOMAL SEX HAVE A DIRECT EFFECT ON LONGEVITY? It has been
suggested that having two X chromosomes offers a direct female longevity advantage (Montagu, 1974) and this possibility resurfaces from time to time. The
author and a colleague (Smith and Warner, 1989) have recently reviewed this
possibility, and it is not the intention to repeat the review here, but only to
summarize its arguments. The term *direct* is used to distinguish primary genetic
effects of the second X chromosome from secondary effects acting, for example,
through sex hormones.

X chromosome inactivation early in development to achieve dosage for X
linked genes similar to that in men would seem to negate much of the potential
advantage to women of having two X chromosomes (Lyon, 1972; Gartler and
Riggs, 1983). There is, however, some residual advantage to the female phenotypic hemizygous mosaic for X-linked genes in the case of heterozygotes for
some X-linked genetic diseases. Some cells in the mosaic can compensate for
genetic deficiencies of others. As described in the context of the prenatal male
die-off, this advantage involves few deaths and does not account for much of the
gender gap. In the female heterozygote for hemophilia only a fraction of the liver
cells can produce clotting factor VIII, but it is active in the blood where enough
is present that the blood clots adequately. In heterozygotes for a deficiency in the
enzyme hypoxanthine phosphoribosyl-transferase, cell selection occurs so that
all red and white blood cell precursors have the X chromosome active that
expresses the intact allele. This purine scavenging enzyme has a predictable
value in nucleic acid biosynthesis that occurs at a rapid rate in the bone marrow
precursors of red and white blood cells. In men the mutation of the single X
chromosome results in the Lesch–Nyhan syndrome (Lyon, 1972; Stout and
Caskey, 1985).

Another beneficial consequence of cell selection in heterozygotes for a genetic
immunodeficiency disease was described.

There is recent evidence for the reactivation of X-linked alleles in female mice
late in life (Cattanach, 1974; Holliday, 1987b; Wareham et al., 1987). In one
study it was shown that the gene for a histochemically recognizable form of the
enzyme ornithine transcarbamylase was activated in about 3 percent of liver cells

in mice 14 to 17 months old. The study raises questions about how much of the X chromosomal gene content is reactivated, whether reactivation occurs in an even larger percentage of cells in older mice (the 14- to 17-month-old mice studied were far from the maximum life span for the strain used), and whether reactivation occurs in other species including humans. Studies by Migeon and co-workers (1988) suggest that X chromosome reactivation may be a very limited process. They found that the X-linked gene for the enzyme hypoxanthine phosphoribosyl-transferase is not spontaneously reactivated with age in human skin fibroblasts from female heterozygotes for the Lesch–Nyhan syndrome.

There is also uncertainty concerning the effects of X-chromosome reactivation. New genetic information could be made available, in the form of both increased gene dosage and previously inactivated alleles. On one hand, aging and mortality could be consequences of limited gene expression. On the other hand, they could be consequences of aberrant gene expression (Cutler, 1985) as is suggested by some evidence of derepression of genes in older cells. Reactivation of genes involved in immune responses could strengthen these responses in elderly women. The gene for the core protein of DNA polymerase-alpha, which is the principal polymerase of DNA synthesis for cellular proliferation, maps to the X chromosome (Smith and Warner, 1989). If impaired cellular proliferation with age plays a role in mortality (see Chapter 3), the activation of this gene could offer a proliferative advantage. A proliferative advantage in cells involved in immune responses could strengthen immune function in women late in life. In the case of genes concerned with cell proliferation, a proliferative advantage in a few stem cells would be quickly amplified because cell selection would operate, and these cells would soon overgrow those without the proliferative advantage provided by the reactivated gene.

Although reactivation would make additional genetic information available, this could be beneficial, or it could be deleterious, with likely gene-specific variations. The new genetic information has the potential to introduce gene dosage imbalance late in life. Gene dosage imbalance is not always deleterious, however, as seen in early embryonic life before X chromosome inactivation. On the other hand, there is an increased variety of gene expression late in life (Cutler, 1985), which could be caused by gene dosage imbalance, and is thought to be deleterious.

Thus, although it is unknown today if the female karyotype of two X chromosomes makes a contribution to the gender gap, findings of modern molecular biology continue to fuel speculation.

There are two early and fragmentary pieces of information that suggest that there may be determinants of longevity on the Y chromosome that contribute to a male disadvantage.

1. A paper from the former Soviet Union (Kuznetsova, 1987) correlates more heterochromatin in the long arm of the Y chromosome with greater male longevity. The genetic content of this DNA is unknown. Considerable heterogeneity has long been recognized in the Y chromosome (Sandberg, 1985), although it was not possible in other studies to correlate the Y-chromosome differences with anything else. This has been taken as evidence for the genetic unimportance of much of the Y chromosome, but the correlation with longevity by Kuznetsova appears to be an exception.

2. Another interesting fragment was presented at the 1987 National Institutes of Health Conference on Gender and Longevity by K.D. Smith (Johns Hopkins) in the description of an Amish family with a deletion in the distal part of the long arm of the Y chromosome (Kunkel et al., 1977) and a record of average male longevity (82.3 years) that exceeds that of other men, Amish men, and even women in the United States.

There are many possible interpretations for these findings. It is not inconsistent that both deleted and added DNA could affect the expression of some genetic determinant of longevity located on the long arm of the Y chromosome. Because the changes do not involve the juxtacentromeric region of the Y chromosome where, as described, deletions are known to affect testicular differentiation, it is unlikely that the effects of the Y chromosome modifications on longevity could involve male sex hormones.

## The Sex and Longevity Differential in Lower Animals

It is sometimes stated that the female is the longer-lived sex in most animal species (e.g., Comfort, 1979; Brody and Brock, 1985), and evidence is provided in the form of increasing proportions of females with age in natural populations (Hamilton, 1948). The cascade of sexual development shown in Figure 5-4 is similar in all mammals, including the same chromosomal mechanism of sex determination and its effect on testicular differentiation, similar sex hormones, and similar hormonal effects. One may wonder if there is some universal property of femaleness reflected in a widespread female longevity advantage. The question merits fresh consideration (Smith, 1989).

Chapter 1 distinguishes between survival and longevity and points out that the survival of animals in natural populations is usually far short of the maximum species life span. Some avoidance of predation may result from female behavior patterns. This is seen throughout animal species from male fish that appear in the deeper waters of the spawning grounds earlier, with increased vulnerability to predation (Woodhead, 1978) to male marsupial rats (*Antechinus*) that engage in reproductive behavior that assures virtually total male mortality shortly after mating (Diamond, 1982). This behavior occurs in the presence of high levels of glucocorticoids, as are seen terminally in some animals, but not in humans (see Chapter 3).

As discussed previously in Chapter 2, humans and other animals die with and presumably of very different pathological processes. Only humans die of ischemic heart disease and cerebrovascular disease in large numbers. Although the effect of sex hormones on circulating lipoproteins is similar in humans and in rats and rabbits (Iozzo et al., 1982; Haug et al., 1984), these species do not die of ischemic heart disease, whereas humans do. The handling of cholesterol is much more important in human life spans than in the life spans of other mammals. The same basic pathway of sexual development has very different consequences in different species, depending on the common causes of death of the species. The sex-related longevity differential as it exists in humans seems to be unique to the human species.

Diverse effects of sex on longevity are observed in laboratory animals kept under carefully controlled conditions to the natural limits of their lives. Male Syrian and Chinese hamsters and guinea pigs are longer lived, whereas female gerbils and mastomys are longer lived (Committee for Animal Models for Research on Aging, 1981). It is doubtful, therefore, that there is a universal female advantage in longevity in animals.

Having written this and having maintained the uniqueness of human longevity throughout this volume, however, it is worth noting two observations that suggest that karyotypic sex may have longevity effects that apply to many species.

1. Several inbred strains of laboratory rodents show no differences in male and female longevity, with virtually superimposable survival curves for the two sexes when kept through their natural life spans under laboratory conditions. These include DBA2/J, C3H$_f$/Bd, and BALB/cAnBd$_f$ mice and Sprague-Dawley, Long-Evans, and Fisher 344 rats (Committee on Animal Models for Research on Aging, 1981). A possible explanation may lie in the detailed homology of the chromosome pairs in these inbred strains including the X chromosomes. Allowing for the gene dosage compensation of X chromosome inactivation, it should make no difference whether there is one X chromosome as in the male or two identical X chromosomes as in the female with respect to the genetic information available.

   It should be noted that not all inbred rat strains have indistinguishable male and female longevity. Female mean survival and maximum life span are substantially longer in rats of the WAG-Rij strain (Masoro, 1990).

2. In birds the mechanism of sex determination is the reverse of what it is in mammals. The male has two Z chromosomes and is the homogametic sex (both sex chromosomes of the same kind), and the female has one Z chromosome and one W chromosome and it is heterogametic. The Z chromosome is much larger than the W chromosome (Takagi and Sasaki, 1974). It should be noted that both cytogenetic (Ohno, 1967) and biochemical (Baverstock et al., 1982) evidence indicates that gene dosage compensation does not occur in birds in the form of Z chromosome inactivation. If the homogametic karyotype confers a longevity advantage, then male birds should be the longer lived sex. Although birds die from different causes than humans, and although there are few studies on the life spans of birds kept under controlled conditions, existing studies show that male birds are longer lived (Levi, 1953; Eisner, 1967; Daniels, 1968; Ricklefs, 1973, Köhler, 1981).

### Men Die Younger, But Women Are Sicker

Women live longer, but there is evidence that they have more illness. This pattern begins in the teenage years (Verbrugge, 1985; Verbrugge and Wingard, 1987) and is, therefore, not explained simply by their older age with its chronic illnesses and functional decrements. Although men die younger of ischemic heart disease, cancer, and cerebrovascular disease, women have higher incidences of a variety of chronic conditions that are debilitating but not commonly fatal. These include musculoskeletal conditions, such as arthritis and osteoporosis with its hip and vertebral fractures, and other conditions ranging from bunions to anemia and depression.

Recently evidence has been published (Ayanian and Epstein, 1991; Steingart et al., 1991) that women receive less aggressive medical care than men. Both studies were of patients with coronary heart disease, and the frequency of diagnostic and therapeutic procedures was less in women. Even with stratification for variables such as age and health insurance, female care was less aggressive. Perhaps women would live even longer if they received health care equivalent to men.

### Consequences of the Gender Gap

A primary consequence of the gender gap is the sharply rising ratio of women to men at advancing ages as shown in Figure 5-3. Widows outnumber widowers in the United States by a ratio of more than 5:1 (Bureau of the Census, 1989). The median income of widowers is $19,500 per year compared with the median income of widows of $10,200. The gender gap results in more female loneliness, financial disadvantage, and poor health.

## Conclusions and Persistent Questions
## about the Gender Gap in Longevity

The sex-related longevity differential in humans is well established in most contemporary societies. Women live longer than men, commonly to the extent of 5 to 10 percent of the mean life expectancy at birth. The gender gap in the United States dates back to at least the mid-nineteenth century. Much of the basis of the gender gap can be identified, and it results from differences in male and female biology. There are large sex differences in mortality rates from different major causes of death.

The following questions concerning the gender gap should be raised in concluding this chapter, even if they cannot be answered now.

1. What is happening to the gender gap? As pointed out (Fig. 5-1), in the United States the gender gap in life expectancies at birth peaked in 1975 at 7.8 years and has fallen since to 6.8 years. There are segments of American society in which the gap is smaller, and others in which it is larger. The trend to a smaller gap will probably continue, based on changes in mortality and changes in society, as discussed in Chapter 7. It is likely that the United States of the future will have a larger proportion of old men. On the other hand, it would be unprecedented for the gap to become less than 3.5 to 5.6 years as it is in developed countries like Japan, Greece, and Israel.

2. Are there contributions to the gender gap in addition to sex hormone modulation of cholesterol handling and society/behavior? The discussions on X chromosomes and immune function consider two additional possibilities. Healthier life styles will not make the gap disappear entirely. Testosterone, despite its adverse effects, plays an essential role in human reproduction.

3. Is there an evolutionary basis for the gender gap? Is it somehow beneficial to the human species that women live longer than men, so that the gap arose because of natural selection? What happened during human evolution so that our lives are so long? This is the topic of the next chapter.

# 6

# The Evolution
# of Human Longevity

Again we find that early maturity, the season of reproduction, and longevity are transmitted to corresponding periods of life.

CHARLES DARWIN (1809–1882)
Essay of 1844

The first five chapters of this book have established the dimensions of contemporary human longevity. In most developed countries men have mean life expectancies at birth of 70 to 75 years and women of 75 to 80 years (see Table 5-1). Current life tables for the United States show that about 30% of those born today will survive to age 85 and about 1.5% will survive to age 100, with many more women surviving to the advanced ages (Metropolitan Life, 1987a). The mean life expectancy continues to increase (see Chapter 7). The record of maximum human longevity is 120 years.

Most humans in developed countries die at about the age of the mean life expectancy at birth, having a survival pattern best described by curve C in Figure 1-1. Most die of relatively few diseases, which include ischemic heart disease, cancer, and cerebrovascular disease. There are a few well-recognized biomedical determinants of whether and when these diseases will occur, and there are behavioral and societal influences on longevity. Causes of death of the very elderly are sometimes more obscure.

Although life span can be shortened by diseases and events, each species has an absolute limit to its longevity, as described in Chapter 1. Humans are the longest lived mammals by a factor of about two. It has been a contention of the author since the beginning that the maximum life span is genetically determined. If this is the case, then longevity has been subject to evolution, and the diverse species-characteristic maximum life spans are the results of evolution. There are mutations affecting genetic determinants of longevity, and natural selection acts to favor the survival of bearers of some alleles but not others. Natural selection does not necessarily favor long life, as will be discussed.

### Evolution of Senescence and Mortality

Senescence and mortality are characteristics of many living things and are related, in that the mortality rate increases with age, as described in Chapter 1. They probably evolved more than once, with a variety of mechanisms being involved.

Mortality is seen in most organisms capable of sexual reproduction from diploid protozoans (Smith-Sonneborn, 1987; Finch, 1990) up the phylogenetic tree to include most multicellular organisms. The consequence of mortality is that creatures capable of sexual reproduction cannot indefinitely use the asexual route of cell proliferation (mitosis) for reproduction. Sexual reproduction, with its opportunities for genetic recombination, was selected as the preferable means of reproduction for species that could also reproduce asexually. Mortality assures that there will be some space for newly produced individuals, with their genetic diversity. There is a biological basis for saying that "with sex came death."

Senescence probably first appeared as decrements in which cell doubling time increased and cell cycling slowed as the proliferative limit was approached. This is seen in diploid ciliated protozoans (Smith-Sonneborn, 1987; Finch, 1990), and a possible parallel may be the clonal senescence of somatic cells cultured from many kinds of animals and tissues (Martin, 1977b). As organisms became more complex, other decrements also occurred with age, and therefore, only a small part of human aging can be related to reduced cellular proliferative activity (see Chapter 3).

There is an abundance of literature on the evolution of senescence, which bears on the questions of what evolved and how evolution resulted in the diverse rates and nature of aging in different living things (Charlesworth, 1980; Hayflick, 1985; Cristofalo, 1988; Kirkwood, 1988; Rose, 1991). Theories on aging can be divided into extrinsic—decrements caused by external agents—and intrinsic—internally programmed decrements. Lifetime DNA damage is an example of extrinsic aging. The damaging agents are extrinsic to the DNA and often to the organism of which the DNA is a part. As a major consequence of DNA damage is somatic mutation, the "somatic mutation theory of aging" is based on extrinsic damage. A mechanism has been suggested for the acceleration of genetic damage late in life by mutations affecting the fidelity of nucleic acid synthesis. A mechanism involving an intrinsic mechanism is suggested by the "antagonistic pleiotrophy theory of aging," which states that some genes that may be neutral or even beneficial early in life may become increasingly deleterious in later life.

Extrinsic and intrinsic mechanisms of aging need not be mutually exclusive. The "throw away soma or disposable soma theory of aging" (Kirkwood, 1987, 1988) recognizes decremental changes with age at the molecular, cellular, organ, and organismal levels, as described in Chapter 3, many of which result from external damage. It also recognizes that there can be some repair of the damage and replacement of damaged elements, but that some changes cannot be reversed, that there is more deterioration than repair, and that the net change is downhill. The ultimate result is mortality. The term *somatic maintenance* is used to describe processes of repair and replacement, which are intrinsic. The theory allows for different species life spans, based on different investments in somatic maintenance. As stated in Chapter 3, the correlation of species life spans with DNA repair activity may be an example of somatic maintenance supportive of longevity. The author would add redundancy and "overprogramming" as properties of living things that allow them to withstand time-related damage.

Much of the evolution of senescence and mortality occurred in the absence of long-lived individuals. Whatever its selective value to a species, senescence seldom occurs under the living conditions of most wild animals (see Chapter 1).

## Evolution of Longevity

The evolution of longevity might seem to be the opposite of the evolution of aging. Decrements and diseases of old age develop more slowly, leading to greater maximum species life spans. Whatever genes are involved in the evolution of longevity must allow for the relationship between senescence and mortality.

There are many pockets of longevity in the animal kingdom—long-lived species on evolutionary branches that are not continua to other longevous taxonomic groups, but rather, specialized forms. Lobsters, giant clams, some species of sharks and turtles, eagles, and parrots are such long-lived evolutionary dead ends (Comfort, 1979). Most of the mammalian orders (see Table 1-1) have long-lived genera that represent evolutionary end points derived from shorter lived less specialized forms. Thus, long-lived ungulates (e.g., elephants) are not a step toward the evolution of long-lived primates. The potential for long species life spans arose independently many times in many genomes. Given the diversity of causes of death (see Table 2-2 and the discussion on animal mortality in Chapter 2) as well as the diversity of genomes, it is not likely that the genetic route to greater species life span was the same each time it evolved.

There are several kinds of genes under current discussion that could undergo mutations and lead to greater species life span.

### Gerontogenes

Gerontogenes have been defined as genes that limit the life span (Johnson, 1990). Mutations in gerontogenes should sometimes result in increased life spans, as factors limiting life are inactivated. There is no current example of a completely characterized gerontogene, but there is a candidate based on a mutant of the nematode *Caenorhabditis elegans* in which the mean life span and the maximum survival are increased by about 70 and 110 percent, respectively (Johnson, 1988), compared with parental strains. The mutant gene has been cloned and is being sequenced. The mechanism of its action in prolonging life is not known. It maps close to a temperature-sensitive gene for fecundity, although it appears to represent a different cistron. Presumably gerontogenes will be of widespread occurrence, and as their mechanisms of action are determined, much more will be learned about longevity. A question for speculation is whether the evolution of longevity resulted from mutations in gerontogenes that alter their life-limiting potential or whether it resulted from changes in other genes that then counter the effects of gerontogenes, or both.

*Longevity Assurance Genes*

The term "longevity assurance genes" was first used by Sacher (1978), and interest in such genes has increased recently. At a conference conducted by the National Institute on Aging in 1989, the following were listed as candidates for longevity assurance genes:

DNA repair enzymes
Antioxidant enzymes and enzymes that produce antioxidant compounds
Proteins involved in cholesterol metabolism
The major histocompatibility complex loci
Regulators of cell proliferation including tumor suppressor genes (see Chapter 3)
Regulators of cell differentiation/senescence
Transcription and elongation factors (e.g., Bravo et al., 1987; Ching and Wang, 1990)

Several kinds of processes can be recognized in this list. There are alleles for healthy cholesterol levels and lipoprotein patterns and alleles for immune function that is strong but avoids the aberrations of autoimmune diseases. Tumor suppressor genes and their mutant alleles that allow tumor growth are discussed in Chapter 3 (Sager, 1989). The repair of DNA damage and other macromolecular damage and the prevention of oxidative damage are examples of processes that could increase life span through increased somatic maintenance.

The above categories only hint at the diversity of mechanisms for life span extension that may be found. Mutation of these genes in combination could result in large longevity increases and the range of maximum life spans seen among animals.

## Natural Selection and the Evolution of Longevity

Just as senescence arose genetically in the absence of aged individuals in natural populations, so did longevity evolve in the absence of longevous individuals. No individual lived close to the maximum species life span. Whatever selection occurred during the evolution of longevity, it was not for longevity. Natural selection for species survival is based on the numbers of offspring surviving to reproduce, and the numbers of their offspring. Longevity evolved as a by-product of other characteristics or coincident with other characteristics that lead to species survival.

The life span involves a prereproductive period when reproductive capacity is achieved, a period of reproductive activity, and a postreproductive period that is, in both humans and laboratory rodents, about half of the maximum life span. The evolution of longevity must involve some time in the life span when natural selection can operate, although the effect of longevity is often to prolong postreproductive life (discussed later).

Another problem is how natural selection could act on mutations of genes affecting life span to fix them in the germ plasm of a species. Although dominance and recessiveness of genes must be regarded today as relative, the heterozygote for an allele must be substantially advantaged for it to be selected favorably. Inbreeding among multiple offspring could produce homozygotes for a mutation in a generation, and the homozygote might be advantaged, even if the heterozygotes were not. Inbreeding is common in species that produce large numbers of offspring at once and that do not disperse widely. An alternative possibility is offered by mutations of X-linked genes. The mammalian male, which is hemizygous for the X chromosome, could express this mutation in every cell, and the mammalian female, which is a mosaic of hemizygous cells with respect to the active X chromosome (see Chapter 5), could express this mutation in approximately half of its cells. On the other hand, X-chromosome inactivation probably does not occur in birds (Ohno, 1967; Baverstock et al., 1982) and does not occur in fruit flies. The expression of mutant recessive sex-linked alleles in the homogametic sex is dependent on sex chromosome inactivation.

## Some Correlates of Longevity

As noted in Chapter 1, larger animals tend to be longer lived. This is the case in the mammalian orders. There is also a correlation between longevity and the proportion of the body weight that is brain (Sacher, 1978), sometimes called the index of encephalization. There appears to be a direct relationship between longevity and the investment made in the development of the soma and especially that part of the soma that is central nervous system. Somatic maintenance is in some direct proportion to the investment made in the soma (Kirkwood, 1988). It seems to make no evolutionary sense to develop a creature as large as an elephant or as smart as a human being with the life span of a mouse.

Life histories, as described in Chapter 1, indicate that there are several strategies to reproductive success. A reciprocal relationship between longevity and fecundity is noted widely in the animal kingdom. This is seen within single species in the case of long-lived nematode mutants (Friedman and Johnson, 1988b; Johnson, 1990) and long-lived fruit fly mutants (Rose and Graves, 1989), which have reduced fecundity. The reciprocal relationship between longevity and fecundity is also seen in comparing mammalian species (Promislow and Harvey, 1990) with the small liter sizes usual among large, long-lived species of several mammalian orders. A liter size of one is usual among all primates. The concept of investment in offspring has been introduced to describe strategies of reproductive success, and species with greater investments in offspring have longer lives. Investment in offspring parallels investment in somatic maintenance.

In the case of invertebrates and other animals that provide no care to the offspring, fecundity can be measured as the number of eggs that hatch. With birds and mammals, reproductive success involves a period of parenting, and, as is discussed, parenting is prolonged in primates, and especially in the human species, to a substantial percentage of the life span. Longevity plays a role in reproductive success in some higher animals based on parenting as discussed.

### Life Extension, Food Deprivation, and Possible Mechanisms for Species Survival in Some Rodents

It has been known for more than 50 years that the deprivation of food to laboratory mice (*Mus musculus*) and rats (*Rattus norvegicus*) results in the prolongation of mean survival and maximum life span by up to 50%. The greater the food deprivation, the greater the life prolongation, up to the point that food intake is reduced by more than half compared with *ad libitum* feeding. Growth is slowed, reproductive maturity and reproductive senescence are both delayed, and the appearance of fatal pathological lesions such as tumors and nephrosclerosis is delayed. The development of late life immunodeficiency is delayed, as is the aging of collagen (Holehan and Merry, 1986; Masoro, 1988). The mechanism of life prolongation by food deprivation is not known.

A question about this phenomenon is whether it is of wide occurrence among animals, including perhaps humans, or whether it is limited to a few species including the rodents in which it has been observed.

Harrison and Archer (1988) have recently pointed out that life extension in periods of food shortage would be an effective survival strategy for small rodents, most of which survive less than a year in the wild. Food deprivation not only prolongs life, but perhaps of greater value to species survival, it prolongs reproductive life. The availability of many foods in temperate climates is on an annual cycle, therefore, in times of food shortage, a year of delayed reproduction would have to be survived.

Natural selection would favor the evolution of delayed senescence at times of food shortage for species with reproductive life spans counted in months. It would not be a useful survival strategy for species living for several years.

Harrison and Archer (1988) point out that the longer lived white-footed mouse (*Peromyscus leucopus*) may have evolved greater longevity with a longer reproductive life span as an alternative strategy for surviving food shortages that occur on an annual cycle. As mentioned in Chapter 3, *Peromyscus* has a more active system for repairing ultraviolet-damaged DNA, suggesting that it has a greater investment in somatic maintenance. There is nothing that precludes *Peromyscus* from having both greater longevity and extended longevity in the face of food restriction, but the contrast between the two mouse species has long been of interest to gerontologists (Sacher and Hart, 1978).

Whether food restriction has life prolonging and senescence-delaying effects on Rhesus monkeys is now being studied. It must be a prolonged investigation. Preliminary data from an ongoing five-year study on middle-aged monkeys with a 30 percent dietary restriction compared with those fed ad libitum indicates that they are in better health with lower blood lipids and lower oxygen consumption (Holden, 1990). The study does not yet show that dietary restriction in monkeys leads to life prolongation. The discussion (see Chapter 2) of causes of death of lower primates raises the possibility of greater records in the future of primate maximum life spans resulting from changed living conditions. If food-deprived monkeys appear to live longer or develop senescent changes more slowly, it will be difficult to interpret the results and to attribute them to prolongation of the species' lifespan by dietary restriction rather than by some other change in their living conditions.

The next chapter considers briefly the implications of life prolongation by food restriction for human longevity.

## Primate Evolution and Longevity

As stated, longevity arose many times in animal evolution, and within each mammalian order there is a diversity of life spans (see Table 1-1) with the longer life spans usually in larger and more specialized species. There is a great diversity of life spans, body sizes, and brain sizes in primates, as shown in Table 6-1. We are the primates with the largest brains and the longest species life span, and human longevity will be considered in the context of the longevity of nonhuman primates. (Recall the discussion in Chapter 2 that some maximum primate life-spans may be increased after changed living conditions.)

The earliest primate fossils date from the Paleocene epoch, 60 to 75 million years ago, with prosimian skulls from both Europe and North America. Many more Prosimian skeletal remains date from the Eocene, with forms recognizable as lemur-like, tarsioid, and lorisiform. Anthropoids appeared during the Oligocene, and considerable diversification of anthropoids occurred during the Oligocene and Miocene epochs in both the New and the Old Worlds. Early apes (hominoids) appeared during the Miocene epoch, 12 to 26 million years ago, and during the Pliocene epoch there was further diversification, with some species having skeletal features consistent with human ancestry. During the Pleistocene epoch beginning 2.5 million years ago, hominids emerged as distinct from higher apes. There are skeletal remains of considerable diversity, but leading to features of modern man (Simons, 1968, 1989).

As shown in Table 6-1, each branch of primate taxonomy has longer and shorter lived species. Among prosimians, the brown lemur (*Lemur fulvus*) has a life span of 39 years, four times that of the sportive lemur (*Lepilemur* sp.), and there is a difference in encephalization that is nearly twofold. A striking example of the evolution of longevity is to be found in New World monkeys, with the white-faced capuchin monkey (*Cebus capucinus*) having a maximum life span of 47 years, which is three times as long as the common squirrel monkey (*Saimiri sciureus*). In these two species, however, the index of encephalization is about the same. There is less variety of life spans among the Old World monkeys, and the species differ little in encephalization.

The evolutionary line that would become modern man (the *Hominidae*) diverged from the higher apes (*Pongidae*) only two to three million years ago, as stated above, with the first recognizable hominids (*Australopithecus africanus*) being bipedal creatures with a cranial capacity and inferred brain size similar to that of modern higher apes of 400 to 500 grams. Although the maximum life span of these early hominids is not known, it is reasonable to assume that it was comparable to that of modern higher apes—about 50 years. Thus, it is likely that there has been a doubling of life span concurrent with a threefold increase in encephalization in 2 to 3 million years of evolutionary time, as originally pointed out independently by Cutler (1975) and by Sacher (1975).

Based on the capacities of fossil skulls the hominid brain reached its present size approximately 100,000 years ago. Although we do not know the maximum potential life spans of these hominids, it is possible that the maximum life span of modern man was reached at that time.

**Table 6-1. Primate Characteristics**

| Major Taxonomic Group by Common Name (Genus) | Maximum Life Span (years) | Body Weight (grams) | Brain Weight (grams) | Encephalization Index | Gestation Period (days) | Age at Sexual Maturity (months) |
|---|---|---|---|---|---|---|
| **Prosimians** | | | | | | |
| Lemur (*Lepilemur*) | 8.6 | 915 | 7.6 | 2.53 | 120–150 | 18 |
| Slow Loris (*Nycticebus*) | 13.3 | 800 | 12.5 | 4.32 | 193 | — |
| Tarsier (*Tarsius*) | 13.4 | 125 | 3.6 | 4.19 | 180 | — |
| Lemur (*Lemur*) | 39.8 | 1,400 | 23.3 | 5.92 | 120–135 | 18 |
| **Anthropoids** | | | | | | |
| New World Monkeys (*Cebidae*) | | | | | | |
| Squirrel Monkey (*Saimiri*) | 15.2 | 660 | 24.0 | 9.8 | 160–182 | — |
| Spider Monkey (*Ateles*) | 33.0 | 8,000 | 108 | 9.16 | 139 | — |
| Capuchin Monkey (*Cebus*) | 46.9 | 3,100 | 71 | 10.9 | 180 | — |
| Old World Monkeys (*Circopithecidae*) | | | | | | |
| Macaques (*Macaca*) | 37.1 | 7,800 | 93 | 8.01 | 160–180 | 40–50 |
| Mangabeys (*Cerocebus*) | 32.7 | 7,900 | 104 | 8.89 | — | — |
| Baboons (*Papio*) | 29.8 | 25,000 | 201 | 8.31 | 170 | 42–48 |
| Higher Apes (*Pongidae*) | | | | | | |
| Gorilla (*Gorilla*) | 47.9 | 105,000 | 500 | 8.37 | 251–289 | 72–120 |
| Chimpanzee (*Pan*) | 53.0 | 46,000 | 404 | 11.4 | 225 | — |
| **Hominidae** | | | | | | |
| Modern Man (*Homo sapiens*) | 120 | 65,000 | 1,330 | 30.1 | 270 | 180 |

*Sources:* Baker and Sprott, 1988; Shiveley and Mitchell, 1986a; Shiveley and Mitchell, 1986b; Stephen et al., 1988; Napier and Napier, 1967.

A question is, what evolved? What genetic changes occurred to result in longevity that can exceed 100 years? What does the evolution of longevity have to do with the evolution of large brains? The comparison of modern chimpanzees and modern humans seems to offer the best way to consider the possible events in the evolution of modern man. Although the two species differ greatly in some respects, they are indistinguishable in others. The alpha and beta subunits of hemoglobin have identical amino acid sequences. Other proteins that have been compared have few amino acid differences (Goodman and Lasker, 1975; King and Wilson, 1975). Mutations in the genes for proteins are under great selective pressure.

DNA segments that do not encode proteins are under less selective pressure and show more differences between the species. The comparison of DNA flanking the beta-globin gene showed a 1.6% divergence between humans and chimpanzees (Miyamoto et al., 1988). The comparison of a hypervariable segment of mitochondrial DNA (mtDNA) of the two species showed a 15.1% difference between the base sequences (Vigilant et al., 1991). This was adjusted to a difference of 69.2% based on evidence that many of the sites had undergone more than one mutation. The authors estimate that the two species diverged 4 to 6 million years ago, and estimate a rate of divergence of 11 to 17% per million years.

The arrangement of the genetic information in the two primates differs substantially. Humans have 46 chromosomes and chimpanzees have 48. The nuclei of chimpanzee cells contain 10% more DNA (Chiarelli, 1975), and the chromosomes of the two species have different banding patterns (Stringer and Andrews, 1988). The homology of the chromosomes of the two species has been extensively investigated (e.g., Yunis and Prakash, 1982).

As pointed out, the life spans of primates can be divided into three periods with respect to reproductive activity: a prereproductive period, much of which involves dependence on parents, a period of reproductive maturity, and a period of postreproductive life that follows reproductive senescence. In the case of humans, reproductive senescence occurs in the middle of the maximum life span, with 50 percent or more being postreproductive. There is a clearly defined menopause in human females that occurs during a brief period of a year or two. The events of reproductive senescence are less clearly defined in some nonhuman primates (Schultz, 1968; Bowden, 1984). There is a well-recognized reproductive decline with age, but studies of both captive and wild individuals of several species indicate that offspring are sometimes produced at advanced ages. Bowden provides the example of chimpanzees that have a maximum life span of about 53 years. The oldest known chimpanzee-producing offspring was 38 years, and cyclical reproductive changes have been observed at 48 years. Reproductive senescence occurs earlier in the life spans of Macaques and is better defined

(Graham et al., 1979). As discussed, reproductive senescence occurring in the middle of the life span offers some advantages in the raising of offspring.

### Factors That Could Favor the Selection of Longevity in Human Evolution

The genes leading to greater human longevity compared with higher apes are as obscure as the genes leading to longevity in other organisms. This section, however, concerns selective factors that could have favored the evolution of human longevity.

Why can humans live so long? There are skeletal remains indicating that humans lived into their 50s as long ago as 100,000 years (see Chapter 1), and, in fact, humans succeeded in becoming a dominant life form on earth with a maximum observed life span of 50 to 60 years and with a mean life expectancy at birth that was a fraction of that. The maximum life span may have been like that of modern humans, but it was never approached. The question is, as posed previously, how did longevity evolve in the absence of longevous individuals?

Two characteristics are identified and discussed that could be contributory to the evolution of human longevity. Each of the characteristics is related to the parenting function that, as pointed out earlier, is a reproductive necessity in birds and mammals and is a lengthy function relative to the total life span of primates and particularly of humans.

LIFELONG FITNESS. Fitness can be defined as the potential to approach the maximum species life span while maintaining a high level of function in all systems and of the integrated organism. Reproductive success and longevity were both related to fitness in humans of the past. In a study of eighteenth and nineteenth century American women, a correlation was observed between longevity beyond the menopause and the number of children born alive (Mayr, 1982). Thus late life fitness can include an earlier reproductive advantage that could be subject to natural selection.

In humans the biological need for parenting can continue more than a decade beyond the time of reproductive senescence. Human parenting, even in its most basic form, involves far more than nursing of the young. Fitness involves a degree of overprogramming so that the postreproductive individual is in good condition to provide for parenting of the late-born, and life can continue much longer. Postreproductive parenting is more important to human reproductive success both because the period of parenting of each offspring represents such a substantial percentage of the total human life span, and because the late-born represent a greater percentage of the total reproductive capacity of humans than of most other animals. Enigmatically, reproductive senescence occurs in the middle of the maximum life spans of rodents as well as humans, although parenting of the late born represents a much greater percentage of the human than the rodent life span.

Even in the absence of parenting behavior, fitness has a role in the reproductive success of male animals. Characteristics that allow for successful competition in mating behavior could confer survival advantages continuing into postreproductive life. These characteristics could be inherited and subject to natural selection.

The inverse relationship between longevity and fecundity has been discussed. The fruit fly mutant to greater longevity displays greater fitness by several tests of function but less fecundity (Rose et al., 1984; Rose and Graves, 1989). Fitness with increased longevity but reduced fecundity may be of negative value in the natural selection of fruit flies, but it can be a successful survival strategy in the evolution of long-lived warm-blooded vertebrates.

MATRILINEAL ADVANTAGES RESULTING FROM BEHAVIOR OF LONGEVOUS FE-MALE PRIMATES. The value of grandparenting extends farther back in primate evolution than the human species. In some social species of non-human primates, particularly Macaques, grandparenting confers advantages on the germ lines of long-lived females.

Two behavioral patterns have been observed that have this effect.

1. Elderly females, which continue to occupy positions of status in Macaque tribes, favor their descendents in protection. This applies to offspring including mature males in their struggles for dominance, and it applies to descendents removed by a generation (grandchildren) (Hrdy, 1981; Bowden, 1984). On the other hand, grandparenting has not been observed in chimpanzees (Goodall, 1971).
2. It has been observed that elderly female Macaques interfere with the reproductive behavior of younger unrelated females but not of related females.

These two behavioral patterns, which are well established in primate social behavior, offer advantages to those carrying the germ lines of longevous females, with specific contributions by postreproductive females to the reproductive success of their descendents.

## Evolution of Human Longevity and Human Causes of Death

Evidence is presented in the previous chapters that modern humans exceed the maximum life spans of other animals and die of different causes, but they inevitably die and of causes that are largely unique to the human species. What do the usual causes of human death have to do with the evolution of human longevity? Although survival of the causes of mortality of lower animals had something to do with the evolution of human longevity, one wonders if ischemic heart disease, the common human malignant tumors, and cerebrovascular disease evolved along with human longevity. If they evolved, what were the selective factors? The diseases were not the usual causes of death of the humans even of the recent past. It may be desirable for the human species that individuals not live forever, but it is difficult to see how these diseases might have evolved to serve this end.

To some extent ischemic heart disease is a consequence of the human diet, with the same diet being atherogenic in some other species. It is partly a result of the human genetic control of cholesterol synthesis and handling. These factors may be coupled to the age of the vasculature in elderly people to make it more vulnerable to atherogenesis. Perhaps atherosclerosis might be more common in other species if they lived longer. Similarly, given the age-relatedness of cancer, one wonders if the pattern of human neoplasms might be seen in other species if they lived long enough.

A theme of this book is that functional decrements based on accumulated age-related unrepaired and unreplaced wear and tear and on diseases that are not fatal in younger people may have an increasing role in the mortality of the very elderly. These functional decrements can result in mortality in the face of small challenges to homeostasis that cannot be compensated in older people. They do not represent diseases of mortality, but rather, challenges to the ultimate durability of the human organism.

## Conclusions and Unanswered Questions about the Evolution of Longevity

Maximum species life spans are genetically determined, and the evolution of longer lived species, including the human species, by mutation and natural selection can be envisioned even if the genes are not yet known. The evolution of longevous species occurred many times and probably involved a variety of mechanisms. The story of primate evolution allows for the evolution of human longevity.

In closing this chapter on the evolution of longevity, there are three questions that have not been posed previously that should be considered.

1. Is greater female longevity a species advantage that could have been subject to natural selection?

The number of female individuals of reproductive age determines the ability of a species to reproduce, and male individuals can be regarded as the more expendable sex and perhaps as a drain on the population as they compete for food and habitat with females and with younger individuals. A male/female ratio of unity is not necessary for reproductive success. Many primate social structures are not supportive of elderly males and nondominant male individuals (Maxim, 1979), but this does little to change sex ratios during the reproductive years. Most late-life fitness that follows from an earlier reproductive advantage would be inherited similarly by both sexes. A possible exception would be mutations of sex-linked genes as discussed in Chapter 5. It is unlikely that the human gender gap is a result of a survival strategy based on the natural selection of mutated genes.

2. What is the biological relationship between brain size (encephalization) and longevity?

The emergence of a single species of hominids worldwide and the disappearance of earlier hominids suggests that competition has permitted the natural selection and survival of only one hominid from among several that were similar and probably occupied similar niches. Evidence would suggest that the selection of the surviving hominid was, probably more than once, based on encephalization with its behavioral advantages. The human evolution of the past 100,000 years, however, could not have been based on encephalization in the face of skeletal evidence that the brain size of modern hominids was reached at that time.

3. Is longevity still evolving in the human species?

As described, the maximum human life span evolved in the absence of humans living this long, but its evolution could have been based on some reproductive advantages of long-lived individuals. It is doubtful that evolution based on reproductive advantage can occur now in developed countries where the number of offspring is small because of birth control, where almost everyone lives well into postreproductive life, and where the survival of offspring usually does not depend on parental longevity. Perhaps it can still occur in less-developed countries where death in the prereproductive and reproductive years is reasonably common and where birth control is less widely practiced. In the absence of a reproductive advantage, what other factors could affect the evolution of human longevity?

Whether or not human longevity will continue to evolve, there are trends that indicate that humans in both developed and in developing countries will live longer in the future. These trends and their implications are discussed in the next chapter.

# 7

# Human Longevity
# in the Future

Do not try to live forever. You will not succeed.

GEORGE BERNARD SHAW (1856–1950)
From *Preface on Doctors, The Doctor's Dilemma*

Human longevity continues to increase. As described in Chapter 1, in this century we have seen about 25 years added to the mean life expectancy at birth in the United States, and in the last two centuries about 40 years have been added, with more than a doubling of the mean life expectancy at birth since 1800. Other chapters have explained these changes, which have resulted from changed risks and changes in the handling of risks. Most of the population lives to much older ages and dies of different causes than in the past.

What can we expect of human longevity in the foreseeable future? There are two approaches to this question that are taken in this chapter. One is to anticipate continuing changes in mean life expectancy as it approaches the maximum human life span as it is known today. The other is to consider possible changes in the maximum life span.

## Recent Changes in Mean Human Life Expectancies

Table 7-1 shows changes during the past 20 to 25 years in life expectancies at birth of several national populations. The limitations of mean life expectancies at birth in describing the longevity of large groups have been discussed previously (see Chapter 1), but the figures can be compared and provide useful indications of changes. The data in Table 7-1 were obtained from the *Demographic Yearbook* of 1979, which includes a review of life expectancies since the 1950s and of 1988, which provides reasonably current values (United Nations, 1979, 1988). The data are self-reported by the countries. The values in the table were selected because they are reasonably comparable in providing values for the early 1960s,

**Table 7-1.   Mean Life Expectancies at Birth,
Selected National Populations, Approximately 1960–1965,
1970–1975, and 1980–1985**

| Country | Years | Mean Life Expectancy at Birth (years) Men | Women |
|---|---|---|---|
| Africa | | | |
| Algeria | 1960–1965 | 47.3 | 49.4 |
| | 1970–1975 | 52.9 | 55.0 |
| | 1983 | 61.6 | 63.3 |
| Congo | 1960–1965 | 36.9 | 40.1 |
| | 1970–1975 | 41.9 | 45.1 |
| | 1980–1985 | 44.9 | 48.1 |
| Ethiopia | 1960–1965 | 35.0 | 38.1 |
| | 1970–1975 | 37.0 | 40.1 |
| | 1980–1985 | 39.3 | 42.5 |
| Nigeria | 1960–1965 | 38.5 | 41.6 |
| | 1970–1975 | 43.4 | 46.6 |
| | 1980–1985 | 46.9 | 50.2 |
| Sierra Leone | 1960–1965 | 36.9 | 40.0 |
| | 1970–1975 | 41.8 | 45.0 |
| | 1980–1985 | 32.5 | 35.5 |
| Zambia | 1960–1965 | 39.4 | 42.5 |
| | 1970–1975 | 44.3 | 47.5 |
| | 1980–1985 | 49.6 | 53.1 |
| North America | | | |
| Canada | 1960–1965 | 68.3 | 74.2 |
| | 1970–1975 | 69.3 | 76.4 |
| | 1980–1985 | 71.2 | 79.0 |
| Guatamala | 1963–1965 | 48.3 | 49.7 |
| | 1970–1975 | 53.7 | 55.5 |
| | 1980 | 55.1 | 59.4 |
| United States | 1965 | 66.8 | 73.7 |
| | 1975 | 68.7 | 76.5 |
| | 1984 | 71.2 | 78.2 |
| South America | | | |
| Bolivia | 1960–1965 | 41.9 | 46.3 |
| | 1970–1975 | 46.5 | 51.1 |
| | 1980–1985 | 48.6 | 53.0 |
| Peru | 1960–1965 | 52.6 | 55.5 |
| | 1970–1975 | 53.3 | 55.9 |
| | 1980–1985 | 56.8 | 60.5 |

(*continued*)

**Table 7-1.** (*continued*)

| Country | Years | Mean Life Expectancy at Birth (years) | |
|---------|-------|------|-------|
| | | Men | Women |
| Asia | | | |
| Afganistan | 1960–1965 | 34.9 | 35.6 |
| | 1970–1975 | 39.9 | 40.7 |
| | 1980–1985 | 36.6 | 37.3 |
| China | 1960–1965 | 53.4 | 56.7 |
| | 1970–1975 | 60.7 | 64.4 |
| | 1980–1985 | 66.7 | 68.9 |
| Japan | 1965 | 67.7 | 72.3 |
| | 1975 | 71.8 | 77.0 |
| | 1985 | 74.8 | 80.5 |
| Philippines | 1960–1965 | 51.0 | 54.1 |
| | 1970–1975 | 56.9 | 60.6 |
| | 1980–1985 | 60.2 | 63.7 |
| Europe | | | |
| Czechoslovakia | 1964 | 67.8 | 73.6 |
| | 1972 | 67.0 | 73.6 |
| | 1984 | 67.1 | 74.3 |
| German Democratic Republic | 1963–1964 | 68.3 | 73.3 |
| | 1976 | 68.8 | 74.4 |
| | 1985 | 69.5 | 75.4 |
| Netherlands | 1961–1965 | 71.1 | 75.9 |
| | 1975 | 71.4 | 77.6 |
| | 1984–1985 | 72.9 | 79.7 |
| Sweden | 1961–1965 | 71.6 | 75.7 |
| | 1971–1975 | 72.1 | 77.7 |
| | 1985 | 73.8 | 79.7 |
| United Kingdom (England and Wales) | 1961–1963 | 68.0 | 73.9 |
| | 1974–1976 | 69.0 | 75.2 |
| | 1983–1985 | 71.8 | 77.7 |
| U.S.S.R. (former) | 1963–1964 | 66.0 | 73.0 |
| | 1971–1972 | 64.0 | 74.0 |
| | 1984–1985 | 62.9 | 72.7 |
| Oceania | | | |
| New Zealand | 1960–1962 | 68.4 | 73.8 |
| | 1970–1972 | 68.6 | 74.6 |
| | 1985 | 71.0 | 76.8 |

*Sources*: United Nations, 1979, 1988.

the early 1970s, and the early to middle 1980s. Separate life expectancy values are given in the table for men and women because they usually differ considerably (see Chapter 5).

In developed countries three patterns of longevity changes can be recognized from the examples in Table 7-1. (a) There are countries in which life expectancies, especially for men, have changed little (less than two years) over the 20 to 25 years considered. These include countries of Eastern Europe, such as Czechoslovakia, and also countries in Western Europe such as the Netherlands. In the Netherlands, male life expectancy changed little, but female life expectancy increased substantially, thus increasing the gender-related longevity differential. (b) There are countries where mean life expectancies for men increased by more than two years during the period considered. Life expectancies for women usually increased more than for men in these countries too. The life expectancy increases in the United States were 4.4 years for men and 4.5 years for women during this period and are relatively large compared with other developed countries. Moreover, life expectancies have continued to increase in the United States since the 1984 values shown in the table to current (1990) values of 72.0 and 78.8 years for men and women respectively (Metropolitan Life, 1992). Smaller (but more than two year) increases in male life expectancy were noted in Canada, the United Kingdom, and Sweden. The greatest increases for mean life expectancy at birth were in Japan where they were 7.1 years for men and 8.2 years for women in the period shown. (c) Then there is the former Soviet Union where self-reported data indicate declines of life expectancies by 3.1 years for men and 0.3 years for women during the period considered, with the gender gap in longevities increasing to 10 years (see Chapter 5).

In less-developed countries there is a common pattern of large increases in mean life expectancies at birth for both sexes during the 20- to 25-year period considered, with the increases ranging from 7 up to 15 years. Life expectancies in the 30s and 40s in the early 1960s are now in the 50s and 60s, although these national populations still do not have life expectancies as long as those of the developed countries. Effective treatment of infectious diseases and reduced infant and childhood mortality (see Chapter 2) explain much of the increased life expectancies in these countries. The changes are similar to those in developed countries during the early decades of this century.

There are a few developing countries where life expectancies changed little (e.g., Afghanistan) or where they actually decreased (e.g., Sierra Leone) during the period shown. Some are countries where the population has had to live under wartime conditions, and some are countries that have become poorer during this period.

It must be concluded that the mean life expectancies of most but not all national populations are increasing. As larger percentages of national populations survive the causes of death of younger people and reach older ages, predictably, most of these older people will die of heart diseases, cancer, and cerebrovascular disease.

## Changing Death Rates from Heart Diseases and Strokes in the United States

As discussed previously (see Chapter 1), recent increases in life expectancy in developed countries have occurred chiefly because of the prolongation of life of the elderly. Mortality rates in the older years have fallen. In the United States this has been chiefly because mortality rates from heart diseases and cerebrovascular disease have fallen during the last 20 to 25 years.

These declines are well-recognized by cardiologists and epidemiologists, but are less well-recognized by other members of the medical profession and by the nonmedical public. The rates to be discussed are age adjusted, therefore, they can be compared over time, although the age structures of the populations are changing. Changes in crude mortality rates from these causes are less striking than age-adjusted rates (Metropolitan Life, 1989b).

Age-adjusted rates for major heart diseases and for ischemic heart disease for men and women combined in the United States from 1965 to 1987 are shown in Figure 7-1. Age-adjusted death rates for ischemic heart disease were not reported in *Vital Statistics of the United States* until 1979, which is why rates for both major and ischemic heart disease since 1979 are shown, and they have declined in parallel. The data show a reduction in the mortality rate from major heart diseases of 35 percent from 1965 to 1987 and of 17 percent for ischemic heart disease from 1979 to 1987. The rates for men and women declined approximately in parallel, but the decline was a little greater for men, thus contributing to the reduction in the gender differential in longevity as observed since 1975 (National Center for Health Statistics, 1965–1988; Metropolitan Life, 1989a). The declining rates show no tendency to taper off up to the present. The declining age-adjusted mortality rates are indicative of delayed mortality from ischemic heart disease rather than its elimination as a cause of death.

Some of the decline has been attributed to a decline in incidence of heart disease associated with healthier life styles in which people smoke less, eat diets with less cholesterol and fat, and exercise more. Studies have shown significant declines in cholesterol levels during the 1980s (e.g. Burke et al., 1991). Some of the decline is because of medical advances ameliorating established heart disease, including the effective treatment of hypertension, coronary bypass surgery,

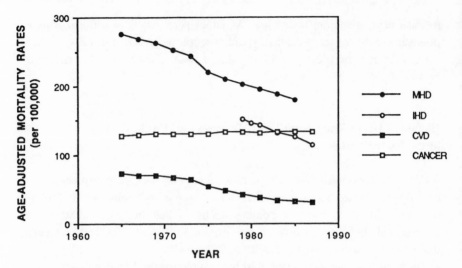

**Figure 7-1.** Mortality rates for major causes of death from 1965 to 1987. Age-adjusted mortality rates for major heart diseases (MHD), ischemic heart disease (IHD), cerebrovascular disease (CVD), and cancer are shown. There have been large rate decreases for the diseases of vascular origin during the period, whereas the death rate from cancer remains unchanged. (Sources: National Center for Health Statistics, 1965–1988.)

and cardiac pacemakers. Some is because of improved survival of patients after heart attacks with interventions such as clot-dissolving agents (Levy, 1981; Goldman and Cook, 1984).

The declining mortality rate from heart diseases in the United States has not been paralleled in most other developed countries. In fact, as will be discussed, the age-adjusted mortality rates from coronary heart disease have increased in some countries during the period of decline in the United States (Levy, 1981). (The term coronary heart disease, as defined in Chapter 2, is used in this section because it is used in Levy (1981), which is the principal reference.) In the 1950s and early 1960s the age-adjusted mortality rate from coronary heart disease in the United States climbed about 10% compared with the 1940s. Except for Finland, it was the highest mortality rate from this cause of any country in the world. It was not until the middle 1970s that the age-adjusted mortality rate from coronary heart disease in the United States fell below the rate in 1940 (Levy, 1981). During the period from 1969 to 1977 the age-adjusted mortality rate from coronary heart disease fell by 22.6%. During this same period, rates in Australia, Canada, and Israel, which were also high, fell between 10 and 20%. The mortality rate in Japan, which was the lowest among developed countries in 1969, fell 19% by 1977, making it still lower relative to most other countries. Mortality rates in Poland, Bulgaria, Romania, and Yugoslavia, however, increased by more than 20% between 1969 and 1977. Rates changed little in most of the countries of Western Europe between 1969 and 1977, including Belgium, the Netherlands, the United Kingdom, and Italy. They also changed little in Finland, which continued to have the highest mortality rate from coronary heart disease for men 35 to 74 in 1977. Thus, the United States has been catching up to other developed countries in achieving a lower mortality rate from coronary heart disease. This is reflected in the greater increase in male life expectancy in the United States compared with most other developed countries. Japan can be considered as a target population in its low age-adjusted mortality rate from coronary heart disease. Will this rate be achieved by other national populations?

An even greater decline in age-adjusted mortality rate from cerebrovascular disease has been observed in the United States, as shown in Figure 7-1. There has been a decline between 1965 and 1987 of nearly 60 percent for the total population, with similar declines for each sex (Metropolitan Life 1989c). Cerebrovascular disease is subject to the same risk factors as coronary heart disease, with hypertension being of even greater relative importance. The effective medical treatment of hypertension has clearly contributed to the decline. The contributions of other factors, including improved management of cases of strokes so that these patients are less likely to die, however, are not clear.

In contrast to heart disease and strokes, the age-adjusted death rate from all malignant tumors combined has remained quite constant or has even increased slightly during the 1965 to 1987 period, as shown in Figure 7-1. The death rate for all malignant tumors combined does not reflect changes in rates from specific kinds of cancer (Marshall, 1990). For example, the mortality rate from malignant melanoma has increased while mortality rates from cancer of the uterine cervix and of the stomach have declined. Questions of age-adjustment methods, changed means of detection, and changed exposure to etiological agents enter into the controversy about what is happening to cancer death rates.

The constancy of the death rate for all cancers combined occurred during a period when cigarette smoking decreased markedly (see Chapter 4), although probably before the benefits of reduced smoking could become fully apparent. There is some evidence that the age-adjusted death rate from lung cancer has peaked and that it may have decreased measurably (Horm and Kessler, 1986), but this has not yet affected the overall age-adjusted cancer mortality rate.

## Projections of Life Expectancy for the Foreseeable Future

Many projections of population size and age structure and of life expectancy in the past have been far from what actually happened. Before 1970 the errors were generally because of the inability to predict fertility changes (living offspring per

woman of child-bearing age). Who could, for example, have predicted the large
drop in fertility that occurred during the Great Depression or the increased
fertility in the Baby Boom years of the 1950s and early 1960s years in advance
(Guralnick et al., 1988; Olshansky, 1988). Extrapolation from current rates and
targeting based on observations of other populations, the principal tools of the
actuary, gave no clues as to the changes that would occur based on events that
were not clearly anticipated. More recently the inaccuracies of actuarial predictions have resulted from erroneous assumptions about mortality. Given the rapid
changes in mortality rates that have occurred in the United States and the incom-
plete understanding of the reasons for their occurrence, it is not surprising that
actual declines in mortality rates outstripped projections.

The Office of the Actuary of the United States Social Security Administration
revises its projections frequently, as reviewed by Olshansky (1988). The most

**Table 7-2A. Life Expectancy at Birth
in the United States**

| Year | Life Expectancies as Calculated for Year | |
| | Men | Women |
| --- | --- | --- |
| 1900 | 47.9 | 50.9 |
| 1930 | 58.0 | 61.3 |
| 1950 | 65.6 | 71.1 |
| 1970 | 67.1 | 74.9 |
| 1980 | 69.9 | 77.5 |
| 1988 | 71.4 | 78.3 |

*Source*: Wade, 1989.

**Table 7-2B.   Projected Life Expectancies in the United States**

| | Alternative I | | Alternative II | | Alternative III | |
| | Men | Women | Men | Women | Men | Women |
| --- | --- | --- | --- | --- | --- | --- |
| 2000 | 72.8 | 79.1 | 72.7 | 80.1 | 72.0 | 80.7 |
| 2010 | 73.2 | 79.5 | 74.1 | 80.8 | 75.0 | 82.3 |
| 2020 | 73.5 | 79.7 | 74.6 | 81.4 | 76.5 | 83.4 |
| 2030 | 73.8 | 80.0 | 75.2 | 82.0 | 77.4 | 84.5 |
| 2040 | 74.1 | 80.3 | 75.7 | 82.6 | 78.4 | 85.5 |
| 2050 | 74.4 | 80.6 | 76.3 | 83.1 | 79.3 | 86.5 |
| 2060 | 74.7 | 80.8 | 76.8 | 83.6 | 80.3 | 87.6 |
| 2070 | 75.0 | 81.1 | 77.3 | 84.2 | 81.3 | 88.6 |
| 2080 | 75.3 | 81.3 | 77.8 | 84.7 | 82.3 | 89.6 |

*Source*: Wade, 1989.

**Table 7-3A.  Life Expectancy at Age 65 in the United States**

|  | Life Expectancies as Calculated for Year | |
|---|---|---|
| Year | Men | Women |
| 1900 | 11.3 | 12.0 |
| 1930 | 11.8 | 12.9 |
| 1950 | 12.8 | 15.1 |
| 1970 | 13.1 | 17.1 |
| 1980 | 14.0 | 18.4 |
| 1988 | 14.9 | 18.8 |

*Source*: Wade, 1989.

**Table 7-3B.  Projected Life Expectancies at Age 65 in the United States**

|  | Alternative I | | Alternative II | | Alternative III | |
|---|---|---|---|---|---|---|
|  | Men | Women | Men | Women | Men | Women |
| 2000 | 15.0 | 18.9 | 15.6 | 19.6 | 16.2 | 20.0 |
| 2010 | 15.2 | 19.0 | 16.0 | 20.1 | 17.0 | 21.2 |
| 2020 | 15.3 | 19.2 | 16.4 | 20.5 | 17.8 | 22.0 |
| 2030 | 15.5 | 19.4 | 16.8 | 20.9 | 18.6 | 22.9 |
| 2040 | 15.7 | 19.6 | 17.1 | 21.4 | 19.3 | 23.7 |
| 2050 | 15.9 | 19.8 | 17.5 | 21.8 | 20.1 | 24.5 |
| 2060 | 16.0 | 20.0 | 17.8 | 22.2 | 20.9 | 25.4 |
| 2070 | 16.2 | 20.2 | 18.2 | 22.6 | 21.7 | 26.2 |
| 2080 | 16.3 | 20.3 | 18.5 | 23.0 | 22.5 | 27.0 |

*Source*: Wade, 1989.

recent revision (Wade, 1989) was made in 1989, based on extrapolation from current data and targeting and modified by what is described as "expert opinion" as to fertility and mortality changes. The analysis of mortality is based on consideration of 10 separate disease categories. In recent years three alternative projections have been offered, representing low, medium, and high estimates of life expectancy through the year 2080. The 1989 mean life expectancies are shown in Tables 7-2 (birth) and 7-3 (age 65). Parts A show life expectancies going back to 1900, and Parts B show projected life expectancies through 2080. It can be noted that most of the projected increased life expectancies are attributable to postponed mortality in the elderly years and decreased mortality rates in the elderly population. One can argue with each of the alternative projections. For example, alternative I indicates a substantial decrease in the present rate of decline of mortality rates. Alternative III projects a small increase in the gender gap in longevities, which is contrary to the present pattern of decrease. Each of the alternative projections shows increased life expectancy. Alternative III anticipates a medical advance that causes a large decrease in the mortality rate during the period of the projection, but the nature of this advance is not described.

The projections all indicate increasing percentages of elderly people in the United States and increasing mean ages of the population. The mean age of the U.S. population in 1988 was 32.1 years. According to the projections of alternative I, this will increase to 37.6 years in 2040 when the Baby Boom population has aged, and it will fall marginally to 37.1 years in 2080. According to the projections of alternative II, the mean ages of the U.S. population will be 41.8 years in 2040 and 42.6 years in 2080. According to alternative III, the mean ages of the population will be 46.6 and 50.6 years, respectively. The projections of mean age require assumptions about fertility and immigration as well as mortality.

As stated previously, the population of the United States now contains 2.5 million people over 85 and about 30,000 centenarians. There are not more very old people today because cohorts were relatively small around 1900 and because many of the people born then succumbed at young ages to diseases that are no longer major causes of death. Projections indicate that there may be 13 million people 85 years and over by 2040 and that there may be a million Americans 100 and over by 2050 and nearly two million by 2080 (Metropolitan Life, 1987a; Longino, 1988) (see Tables 7-3A and 7-3B). The chances of reaching 100 have approximately doubled every 10 years in the recent past, with the chances for women being about four times those for men.

These projections all involve increases in mean life expectancy without any change in the maximum potential life span of the human species. They are based on declining mortality rates from known causes of death and on postponed mortality rather than on the elimination of causes of death.

### Further Reductions in Mortality Rates from Vascular Diseases That Can be Anticipated

As shown in Figure 7-1, the declines in age-adjusted death rates from ischemic heart disease and cerebrovascular disease, which are not fully understood, continue without any sign of leveling off. As later cohorts age that have smoked less, eaten better, exercised more, and are generally better educated and more prosperous, there is reason to expect them to live longer and continue the trends of greater longevity and of declining mortality rates from vascular diseases.

Improved management of hypertension should continue, with its salutary effect on longevity, and there are other pharmacological interventions that have the potential to reduce mortality from heart diseases and strokes. The effects on mortality rates from these interventions are only beginning to be felt.

Among the pharmacological effects of aspirin is a reduction in blood coagulability (clotting). There is recently published evidence that one aspirin tablet (325 mg) every other day reduces the incidence of myocardial infarction in American male physicians by 44 percent compared with a control group (Steering Committee of the Physicians' Health Study Research Group, 1989). Although such a beneficial effect of aspirin on thrombotic ischemic heart disease has been suspected for the past 10 years, most of the decline in the death rate from ischemic heart disease during the 1970s and 1980s occurred without widespread consumption of aspirin for that reason. It should be noted that a British study (Peto et al., 1988) does not agree with the American study and failed to indicate a beneficial effect of aspirin on the rate of myocardial infarcts. It should also be noted that in the American study the use of aspirin was correlated with a small increase in hemorrhagic cerebrovascular disease, although this increase was not statistically significant and was more than offset by the beneficial effects on coronary heart disease. It is likely that increased use of this nonprescription drug will further reduce the mortality rate from myocardial infarcts.

There are several pharmacological interventions that reduce serum cholesterol. These include sequestrants of intestinal bile acids (e.g., cholestyramine) that block the enterohepatic cycling of cholesterol. These sequestrants are resins that bind bile acids in the intestine, preventing their resorption. Increased hepatic cholesterol synthesis to compensate for reduced cholesterol absorption is inhibited by niacin (nicotinic acid, vitamin $B_6$), which is, therefore, often used synergistically with sequestrants (Kane et al., 1981).

There are competitive inhibitors of 3-hydroxy-3-methylglutaryl-coenzyme A reductase, the enzyme that is limiting in hepatic cholesterol synthesis (e.g., lovastatin). It is possible to reduce serum cholesterol and low-density lipoprotein cholesterol by 30 to 50 percent (Grundy, 1988). These reductions are far greater than can be achieved by the reduced intake of dietary cholesterol and lipids (Goldman and Cook, 1984). As these drugs must be taken on a prolonged and possibly lifetime basis, they are not now being recommended for the population as a whole, but only in cases of hypercholesterolemia. They have the potential to lower further the death rate from ischemic heart disease, and improved coronary circulation has been observed after they have been used (Brown et al., 1990).

Hyperlipidemia is also a risk factor in cerebrovascular disease, and these medications may be expected to lower stroke mortality further as well as mortality from ischemic heart disease.

Olshansky and colleagues (1990) have recently calculated that even if mortality rates from ischemic heart disease, cancer, strokes, and diabetes could be reduced by 75 percent in the United States, the mean life expectancy at birth would be extended only to about 85 years. A life expectancy at birth of 85 years would mean an average age at death of 86 years for men and of 91 for women.

They demonstrate that at this point large changes in mortality rates have a small impact on the life expectancy and argue that life expectancy is an ever less useful concept in describing developed societies. If mortality from these diseases could be eliminated completely, mean life expectancy at birth would be extended only to about 90 years. Interestingly the alternative III projections by the Office of the Actuary of the Social Security Administration lead to a mean life expectancy in 2080 (Wade, 1989) that approaches the number calculated by Olshansky and colleagues (1990). This conclusion was reached by a different process than used by Olshansky and colleagues, and it will be recalled that alternative III required unspecified major medical advances that would reduce mortality rates. Elderly people will continue to die under these circumstances, and causes of death in many cases may be obscure.

### Behavioral and Societal Changes Favoring Increased Life Spans

Whatever one thinks of our species today and in the future, there is evidence of behavioral and societal contributions to recent increases in human life spans. From Chapter 4 on, there are references to healthier life styles and reduced unhealthy behavior, including less smoking. Although some persons have failed to benefit from these changes, and although it can be argued that the trend now is to declines in some economic and social conditions, there is a strong indication that behavioral and societal changes will continue to be supportive of increased human life spans.

### The Possibility of Increasing the Maximum Human Life Span

The changes that have occurred in human life expectancies and in disease-specific mortality rates represent increases in the mean life span but probably not in the maximum life span. The postponement of mortality and the projections of increased life expectancy that have been described are still very much within today's maximum human life span.

The record human longevity of 120 years, as described in Chapter 1, is based on a small number of outlyers compared with the millions of centenarians projected for the next century in the United States and other developed countries. Moreover, as discussed in Chapter 1, many of the very old people of the future will have credible records establishing age and continuing identity. It is likely that the record of 120 years will be exceeded at least marginally within the limits of an unchanged potential maximum human life span.

A few possible interventions have been suggested as prolonging the maximum human life span. These are not interventions to reduce mortality from a single disease or pathological process, but rather interventions which would postpone mortality on a broader biological basis.

## Genetic

In the previous chapter the evolution of human longevity was discussed. An argument was presented that human longevity may have ceased to evolve, and therefore, it may have stopped increasing on the basis of evolution. Although human longevity evolved rather rapidly in evolutionary time, the doubling of human life span compared with that of an ape-like ancestor required two to three million years, and a change in human longevity based on such a rate of evolution is not likely to be detectable in any time period imaginable by most contemporary people. Thus, it is not fruitful to speculate on whether some longer lived humans will evolve someday.

As understanding of the human genome progresses it may become possible to identify genes that could play a role in long human life. In the future it may be interesting to compare what has been learned about longevity genes with the speculation of today (see Chapter 6). Genetic manipulations to produce longer lived humans may someday be a temptation.

A few possible interventions have been suggested as prolonging the maximum human life span without changing the genome.

## Dietary Restriction

Dietary restriction prolongs the mean survival and the maximum life spans of laboratory rodents by about 50 percent, as described in Chapter 6. The phenomenon could be a useful evolutionary adaptation to food scarcity in rodents, with the delay of significance to survival being not so much a delay in mortality as a delay in reproductive senescence (Harrison and Archer, 1988).

It has not been determined whether dietary restriction prolongs the life spans of humans. When one reads predictions in the popular press of maximum potential human life spans ranging up to 180 years, this is speculation based on the possible applicability of the rodent effect to the maximum human life span known today, human longevity, but it is most uncertain that this applicability exists. As pointed out in Chapter 6, the effect of dietary restriction on longevity and reproductive senescence would be useful in the survival of short-lived species, but not of long-lived species. Still, the effect could exist in long-lived species also. If dietary restriction can prolong the maximum human life span, it need not be the same percentage as the prolongation of rodent life spans. The amount and timing of dietary restriction needed for significant life prolongation in humans is uncertain. Dietary restriction at a young age, which causes the greatest prolongation of rodent life, causes not only retarded growth and sexual development, but may also cause mental retardation in humans.

### Other Interventions

A review (Schneider and Reed, 1985) considers several other interventions that could prolong life. Some interventions involve chemicals that act as scavengers of free radicals and appeal to those who believe that unrepaired free radical damage accumulated over the life span is important in aging and mortality. Some compounds that appear to prolong life in rodents cause weight loss and may be working through dietary restriction.

Some interventions involve improvements in immune function and modifications of endocrine function. A recent endocrine intervention is the use of growth hormone in elderly men who have evidence of a deficiency of this hormone (Rudman et al., 1990). Compared with untreated controls there were some body composition changes consisting of a loss of fat and an increase in lean body mass. The changes were suggestive of a reversal of body composition changes that usually occur with age. It is unknown, however, if, for example, the increased lean body mass is reflected in an increase in muscle strength.

It is fair to say that none of these interventions in the present state of development offers much hope for the prolongation of the maximum human life span.

## Consequences of Increased Longevity in Developed Countries

Life expectancies of most national populations have increased and continue to increase, based on well-established trends. The United States of the future will include even larger proportions of elderly people. Those 85 years and over constitute the fastest growing age group of the American population on the basis of percent increase, and this will be accelerated during the first half of the next century by the aging of Baby Boom cohorts.

The prospect of an aging society has been considered extensively by many authors (e.g., Vaupel and Gowan, 1986; Schneider and Guralnick, 1990), and the purpose here is not to review what has been written, but only to discuss a single point in the context of longevity as it has been developed in this volume.

The relationship of aging to disability and to mortality in the future will determine much about the consequences of increasing longevity. Active life expectancy (Manton and Stallard, 1991) is shorter than life expectancy. The very old (85 years and over) of today are 22% institutionalized, although 50% still live independently in their own homes (Longino, 1988). About half are disabled as measured by the inability to perform one or more of the activities of daily living, which include dressing and toileting, or as defined by the inability to use public transportation of six months or more duration (Katz et al., 1983, Manton and Soldo, 1985; Soldo and Manton, 1985). It is estimated that between 20 and 47% have symptoms of dementia (Evans et al., 1989). The very old of today were born in the last years of the nineteenth century and the early years of this century. The mean level of education is 8.6 years. Only 50% have pension incomes. Sixteen percent have family incomes below the poverty level, and 12% are on public assistance.

Although the very old of future cohorts will be better educated and probably more prosperous, will they be in better health? They will be much more numerous, and the age distribution in the population will be toward even more advanced ages than it is today. The "compression of morbidity hypothesis" suggests that they may be healthier (Fries and Crapo 1981; Fries, 1989, 1990). This hypothesis states that as death rates from the major causes of elderly mortality decrease, morbidity from these causes will also decrease. For the compression of morbidity to occur, morbidity must decrease faster than mortality. There is little evidence that this has occurred to the present. Also it must be recognized that much morbidity of the elderly is caused not by the diseases of mortality, but by diseases that are usually chronic but nonfatal such as arthritis, osteoporosis, depression, and dementia. With the population living to greater ages, not only must a cohort reach an elderly age in better condition, but it must maintain a better condition to an even more advanced age if morbidity is to be compressed.

The concept of *healthy aging* (Schmidt, 1989), also called *successful aging* (Rowe and Kahn, 1987), offers some hope that future cohorts will reach advanced ages with less morbidity than is seen today through the avoidance of risks that are associated with morbidity. Healthy aging involves improved health practices early in life so that advanced age is reached with less chronic disease and fewer of the functional decrements associated with aging even without defined diseases. Risks leading to diseases of mortality and morbidity are to be avoided. Smoking is condemned, but, as pointed out, most smokers die at relatively young ages after relatively brief illnesses, and therefore, smoking contributes little to the morbidity or the mortality of the very old. Dementia of the Alzheimer's type increases in incidence with age, but, except for a genetic predisposition associated with a fairly well-defined gene, risks have yet to be identified that may have an effect on the incidence and progress of Alzheimer's disease (Fries, 1990).

Elderly cohorts of the future may be expected to seek better health care, but much late-life morbidity is refractory to the medical interventions of today.

Projections about life expectancy, population age distribution, morbidity, and mortality could be greatly changed by medical and public health practices that could prolong life further. They could also be changed by altered public attitudes concerning the desirability of prolonging the lives of very old people (e.g., Callahan, 1987) and concerning laws and policies about the "right to die."

## Conclusions

Human life expectancy will continue to increase. In developed countries mortality rates from some of the principal diseases of mortality are falling. In most of the less-developed countries the changes that led to longer life in developed countries are underway. It seems likely that the mean life expectancy at birth will be extended by several years over the next decades. Most of the increase will be because of prolongation of the lives of elderly people. Predictably the United States of the future will have an older population with larger percentages of people at advanced ages.

Possible changes in the maximum human life span are subjects for speculation.

# 8

# Human Longevity Seen from the Perspective of This Book

I should regret very much if it were assumed from what I have presented that the span of human life is practically fixed and that no extension of it can be expected beyond the average of sixty-five indicated by my life table.

LOUIS I. DUBLIN
The Possibility of Extending Human Life
Lecture to the Harvey Society, 1922

Some readers may be concluding that the story of human longevity is nearly complete. The human life span has increased, with the first changes being genetic and resulting in a potential species maximum life span that is approximately twice as long as that of the higher apes, which were our ancestors. This potential went unrealized for millennia during prehistoric times and was approached only rarely in early civilizations. It is more commonly approached in modern times as living conditions, public health, and medical care have reached the levels they are today in developed countries. Increased life expectancies have occurred by the postponement of mortality for most people because of reduced mortality rates for diseases that have been the major causes of death. Earlier these were infectious diseases affecting predominantly young people. More recently they have become the fatal diseases of later life—ischemic heart disease, cancer, and strokes. Even today, only a few individuals survive within a decade of the maximum established human life span of 120 years. There remains ample opportunity for further increases in life expectancies within this established maximum, and more increases have been predicted. As more people live to very old ages, what will be their causes of death?

There is still much to be learned about the biomedical determinants of the maximum life span and how they operate. Do they operate by increasing the incidence of fatal diseases late in life? A major theme of this book is that the maximum species life span is genetically determined, but the genes involved are unknown today. Could a failure of genetically based processes required for somatic maintenance to keep pace with age-related wear and tear explain human mortality at ages approaching the maximum life span?

Just as fatal diseases cause mortality for most individuals well short of the maximum human life span, so do behavioral and societal factors act to shorten life. They do so through fatal diseases and violence. There are intriguing correlations between life expectancy and behavioral and societal determinants that are not easily explained.

The predictable future of human longevity is that the mean life expectancy will continue to increase—probably for the next century or more. The increased mean life expectancy at birth that is projected could be a decade longer than it is today in the United States, and it will probably be much more than a decade in those developing countries that are catching up to today's developed countries.

Most of the increase will result from the prolongation of life of elderly people. Age-adjusted mortality rates from cardiovascular and cerebrovascular diseases will continue to fall, providing a basis for much of the increase in life expectancy. National populations may become more like each other as mortality rates decline to target levels represented by populations with the lowest mortality rates. Japan is a target population for its cardiovascular disease mortality rate, but Japanese mortality rates from cerebrovascular diseases and cancer are not especially low.

Even as mortality rates from the fatal diseases of late life decline further, people will continue to die and will not live forever. There is the possibility of death without recognizable fatal disease, and entries on death certificates may increasingly reflect the terminal breakdown of homeostasis. Pneumonia may sometimes be a pathological reflection of breakdown of homeostasis, and it may be listed more frequently in the United States as the cause of death of very old people.

The quotation at the beginning of this chapter is by a predecessor speaking about the future of human longevity 70 years ago. At that time he was impressed by recent changes in the survival of the very young and also by the absence of increased survival of those in later life. The quotation leaves open the possibility that unanticipated changes could occur that would affect human survival profoundly. As subsequent history has proved, such changes did occur. The author wants to subscribe to continuing uncertainty about future changes in human longevity, and it is doubtful that the story of human longevity as it is described here and as it can be anticipated today is complete.

It would be premature, therefore, to discount the possibility that human longevity will increase further because of increases in the maximum life span in addition to increases in the mean life expectancy that fall within the maximum life span as it is known today. Increases in the maximum life span may have a greater effect on longevity than the marginal increases that may be expected as more outlyers reach the limit of today's maximum human life span. Increases in the maximum human life span may be the consequence of interventions or even of modifications in the human genome. On the basis of present understanding of genetic and other determinants of life span it is not known what these interventions and modifications might be, but as the biomedical limits of the maximum life span are better understood, a scientific rationale may emerge. A result might not only be a delay in mortality, but a postponement of some of the characteristics of senescence that precede and predispose to mortality and that cause disability.

# Appendix

**Table A-1.  Life Expectancy in Developed Countries**

| Country and Year | Sex | Life Expectancy at Age | | |
|---|---|---|---|---|
| | | Birth | 1 Year | 65 Years |
| Australia, 1986 | Male | 72.8 | 72.5 | 14.6 |
| | Female | 79.1 | 78.7 | 18.5 |
| Austria, 1987 | Male | 71.5 | 71.3 | 14.2 |
| | Female | 78.1 | 77.8 | 17.4 |
| Belgium, 1979–1982 | Male | 70.0 | 70.0 | 13.0 |
| | Female | 76.8 | 76.6 | 16.9 |
| Bulgaria, 1978–1980 | Male | 68.3 | 69.0 | 12.7 |
| | Female | 73.5 | 74.0 | 14.6 |
| Canada, 1984–1986 | Male | 73.0 | 72.6 | 14.9 |
| | Female | 79.8 | 79.3 | 19.2 |
| Czechoslovakia, 1985 | Male | 67.2 | 67.3 | 11.7 |
| | Female | 74.7 | 74.6 | 14.9 |
| Denmark, 1986–1987 | Male | 71.8 | 71.4 | 14.1 |
| | Female | 77.6 | 77.2 | 17.9 |
| Finland, 1986 | Male | 70.5 | 70.0 | 13.4 |
| | Female | 78.7 | 78.0 | 17.4 |
| France, 1987 | Male | 72.0 | 71.7 | 15.0 |
| | Female | 80.3 | 79.8 | 19.4 |
| Germany (DDR), 1986–1987 | Male | 69.7 | 69.4 | 12.5 |
| | Female | 75.7 | 75.3 | 15.5 |
| Germany (DFR), 1985–1987 | Male | 71.8 | 71.5 | 13.8 |
| | Female | 78.4 | 78.0 | 17.6 |

*(continued)*

**Table A-1.** (*continued*)

| Country and Year | Sex | Life Expectancy at Age | | |
|---|---|---|---|---|
| | | Birth | 1 Year | 65 Years |
| Greece, 1980 | Male | 72.1 | 72.8 | 14.6 |
| | Female | 76.3 | 76.8 | 16.7 |
| Hungary, 1987 | Male | 65.7 | 66.0 | 12.0 |
| | Female | 73.7 | 73.8 | 15.2 |
| Iceland, 1983–1984 | Male | 74.0 | 73.4 | 15.5 |
| | Female | 80.2 | 79.7 | 18.9 |
| Ireland (Republic of), | Male | 71.0 | 70.7 | 12.6 |
| 1985–1987 | Female | 76.7 | 76.3 | 16.2 |
| Israel, 1985 | Male | 73.5 | 73.5 | 15.1 |
| | Female | 77.0 | 76.9 | 16.5 |
| Italy, 1983 | Male | 71.4 | 71.4 | 13.6 |
| | Female | 78.1 | 78.0 | 17.4 |
| Japan, 1987 | Male | 75.6 | 75.0 | 16.1 |
| | Female | 81.4 | 80.8 | 19.7 |
| Luxembourg, 1980– | Male | 70.0 | 68.9 | 12.8 |
| 1982 | Female | 76.7 | 76.6 | 15.1 |
| Netherlands, 1985– | Male | 73.0 | 72.6 | 13.9 |
| 1986 | Female | 79.6 | 79.1 | 18.6 |
| New Zealand, 1986– | Male | 71.0 | 70.9 | 13.7 |
| 1988 | Female | 77.3 | 77.0 | 17.6 |
| Norway, 1987 | Male | 72.8 | 72.4 | 14.4 |
| | Female | 79.5 | 79.1 | 18.5 |
| Poland, 1985 | Male | 66.8 | 67.7 | 12.3 |
| | Female | 75.2 | 75.3 | 15.9 |
| Portugal, 1979–1982 | Male | 68.3 | 69.1 | 13.4 |
| | Female | 75.2 | 75.7 | 16.1 |
| Romania, 1976–1978 | Male | 67.4 | N/D | N/D |
| | Female | 72.2 | | |
| Spain, 1980 | Male | 72.6 | 72.6 | 15.0 |
| | Female | 78.6 | 78.5 | 18.5 |
| Sweden, 1985 | Male | 73.8 | 73.3 | 14.7 |
| | Female | 79.7 | 79.2 | 18.5 |
| Switzerland, 1984– | Male | 73.5 | 73.1 | 15.1 |
| 1985 | Female | 80.0 | 79.5 | 18.9 |
| United Kingdom, | Male | 71.8 | 71.5 | 13.4 |
| 1983–1985 | Female | 77.7 | 77.4 | 17.5 |
| United States, 1986 | Male | 71.3 | 71.1 | 14.7 |
| | Female | 78.3 | 78.0 | 18.6 |
| USSR (former), | Male | 64.1 | 65.0 | 12.3 |
| 1985–1986 | Female | 73.3 | 73.9 | 15.8 |
| Yugoslavia, 1984– | Male | 68.1 | 69.0 | 13.8 |
| 1985 | Female | 73.5 | 74.4 | 16.6 |

*Source*: United Nations, 1990.

**Table A-2. Life Expectancy, Less-Developed Countries**

| Country and Year | Sex | Life Expectancy at Age | | | | |
|---|---|---|---|---|---|---|
| | | Birth | 1 Year | 5 Years | 10 Years | 65 Years |
| Algeria, 1983 | Male | 61.6 | 66.3 | 63.8 | 59.6 | 12.2 |
| | Female | 63.3 | 67.8 | 65.4 | 61.2 | 13.2 |
| Argentina, 1980– 1981 | Male | 65.5 | 67.2 | 63.6 | 58.8 | 12.5 |
| | Female | 72.7 | 74.1 | 70.6 | 65.7 | 16.1 |
| Bangladesh, 1988 | Male | 56.9 | 63.7 | 62.8 | 58.7 | 12.2 |
| | Female | 55.9 | 61.5 | 61.3 | 57.3 | 12.0 |
| Botswana, 1981 | Male | 52.3 | 55.9 | 54.5 | 50.4 | 10.2 |
| | Female | 59.7 | 62.6 | 61.5 | 51.6 | 12.5 |
| Cuba, 1983–1984 | Male | 72.7 | 73.0 | 69.3 | 64.5 | 15.6 |
| | Female | 76.1 | 76.2 | 72.4 | 67.5 | 17.3 |
| Ecuador, 1985 | Male | 63.4 | 67.1 | 64.9 | 60.4 | 14.3 |
| | Female | 67.6 | 70.6 | 68.4 | 63.1 | 15.7 |
| Guatamala, 1979– 1980 | Male | 55.1 | 59.1 | 58.5 | 54.4 | 13.4 |
| | Female | 59.4 | 63.0 | 62.8 | 58.7 | 14.2 |
| India, 1976–1980 | Male | 52.5 | 58.6 | 58.8 | 54.8 | 11.7 |
| | Female | 52.1 | 58.6 | 60.2 | 56.6 | 13.2 |
| Iran, 1976 | Male | 55.8 | 60.8 | 58.4 | 53.9 | 11.6 |
| | Female | 55.0 | 60.1 | 58.7 | 54.4 | 12.2 |
| Malawi, 1977 | Male | 38.1 | 45.8 | 49.4 | 47.4 | 10.6 |
| | Female | 41.2 | 47.9 | 51.5 | 49.8 | 11.4 |
| Mali, 1976 | Male | 46.9 | 53.8 | 59.5 | 56.7 | 14.6 |
| | Female | 49.7 | 55.3 | 60.7 | 57.7 | 16.0 |
| Nepal, 1981 | Male | 50.9 | 56.6 | 55.8 | 51.7 | 11.0 |
| | Female | 48.1 | 54.1 | 54.7 | 51.0 | 11.5 |
| Pakistan, 1976–1978 | Male | 59.0 | 66.5 | 65.2 | 61.3 | 16.1 |
| | Female | 59.2 | 65.6 | 64.8 | 60.7 | 15.7 |
| Rwanda, 1978 | Male | 45.1 | 52.2 | 53.3 | 49.4 | 10.9 |
| | Female | 47.7 | 54.0 | 55.2 | 51.1 | 11.8 |
| Sierra Leone, 1985– 1990 | Male | 39.5 | N/D | N/D | N/D | N/D |
| | Female | 42.6 | N/D | N/D | N/D | N/D |
| Sri Lanka, 1981 | Male | 67.8 | 69.0 | 65.7 | 61.0 | 14.2 |
| | Female | 71.7 | 72.7 | 69.5 | 64.8 | 15.7 |
| Swaziland, 1976 | Male | 42.9 | 50.3 | 51.2 | 47.3 | 10.1 |
| | Female | 49.5 | 56.9 | 57.3 | 53.3 | 12.5 |
| Syria, 1976–1979 | Male | 63.8 | 66.9 | 64.3 | 59.9 | 13.2 |
| | Female | 64.7 | 67.0 | 64.4 | 60.1 | 13.2 |
| Uruguay, 1984–1986 | Male | 68.4 | 69.7 | 65.9 | 61.0 | 13.5 |
| | Female | 74.9 | 75.9 | 72.1 | 67.2 | 17.3 |

*Source*: United Nations, 1990.

**Table A-3. Principal Causes of Death, Developed Nations, 1980s**

| Nation and Year | Death Rate per 100,000 | Principal Causes of Death | Death Rate from Cause per 100,000 | Percentage of Total National Mortality from Cause |
|---|---|---|---|---|
| United States, 1983 | 861 | Ischemic heart disease | 236 | 27 |
| | | Cancer | 189 | 22 |
| | | Other circulatory diseases | 91 | 11 |
| | | Cerebrovascular | 66 | 8 |
| | | Accidents | 39 | 4 |
| | | Ill-defined causes | 13 | 1 |
| Australia, 1984 | 707 | Ischemic heart disease | 199 | 28 |
| | | Cancer | 166 | 23 |
| | | Cerebrovascular | 81 | 11 |
| | | Other circulatory diseases | 50 | 7 |
| | | Ill-defined causes | 5 | <1 |
| Belgium, 1984 | 1,127 | Cancer | 273 | 24 |
| | | Ischemic heart disease | 149 | 13 |
| | | Other circulatory diseases | 138 | 12 |
| | | Accidents | 127 | 11 |
| | | Cerebrovascular | 125 | 11 |
| | | Ill-defined causes | 76 | 7 |
| Canada, 1984 | 699 | Ischemic heart disease | 190 | 27 |
| | | Cancer | 178 | 22 |
| | | Cerebrovascular | 55 | 8 |
| | | Other circulatory diseases | 48 | 7 |
| | | Ill-defined causes | 8 | 1 |
| Czechoslovakia, 1984 | 1,190 | Ischemic heart disease | 287 | 24 |
| | | Cancer | 234 | 20 |
| | | Cerebrovascular | 198 | 17 |
| | | Accidents | 94 | 8 |
| | | Other circulatory diseases | 60 | 5 |
| | | Ill-defined causes | 11 | 1 |
| France, 1984 | 987 | Cancer | 238 | 24 |
| | | Other circulatory diseases | 132 | 13 |
| | | Cerebrovascular | 112 | 12 |
| | | Ischemic heart disease | 96 | 10 |
| | | Accidents | 64 | 6 |
| | | Ill-defined causes | 62 | 6 |
| Greece, 1984 | 893 | Cancer | 178 | 20 |
| | | Cerebrovascular | 172 | 19 |
| | | Other circulatory diseases | 117 | 13 |
| | | Ischemic heart disease | 87 | 10 |
| | | Ill-defined causes | 57 | 6 |
| Japan, 1985 | 623 | Cancer | 155 | 25 |
| | | Cerebrovascular | 112 | 18 |
| | | Other circulatory diseases | 78 | 13 |

(*continued*)

**Table A-3.** (*continued*)

| Nation and Year | Death Rate per 100,000 | Principal Causes of Death | Death Rate from Cause per 100,000 | Percentage of Total National Mortality from Cause |
|---|---|---|---|---|
| | | Accidents | 59 | 9 |
| | | Ischemic heart disease | 41 | 7 |
| | | Ill-defined causes | 25 | 4 |
| Poland, 1985 | 1,025 | Cerebrovascular | 209 | 20 |
| | | Cancer | 180 | 18 |
| | | Other circulatory diseases | 122 | 12 |
| | | Ischemic heart disease | 87 | 8 |
| | | Accidents | 52 | 5 |
| | | Ill-defined causes | 70 | 7 |
| Portugal, 1985 | 958 | Cerebrovascular | 237 | 25 |
| | | Cancer | 158 | 16 |
| | | Ischemic heart disease | 83 | 9 |
| | | Other circulatory diseases | 71 | 7 |
| | | Ill-defined causes | 109 | 11 |
| Romania, 1984 | 1,033 | Cerebrovascular | 153 | 15 |
| | | Ischemic heart disease | 148 | 14 |
| | | Other circulatory diseases | 141 | 14 |
| | | Cancer | 128 | 12 |
| | | Hypertension | 85 | 8 |
| | | Ill-defined causes | 0.5 | <1 |
| Sweden, 1985 | 1,126 | Ischemic heart disease | 379 | 34 |
| | | Cancer | 236 | 21 |
| | | Cerebrovascular | 116 | 10 |
| | | Other heart disease | 57 | 5 |
| | | Accidents | 33 | 3 |
| | | Ill-defined causes | 9 | <1 |
| United Kingdom, 1984 | 1,139 | Ischemic heart disease | 316 | 28 |
| | | Cancer | 278 | 24 |
| | | Cerebrovascular | 144 | 13 |
| | | Other circulatory diseases | 71 | 6 |
| | | Accidents | 25 | 2 |
| | | Ill-defined causes | 5 | <1 |

*Source*: United Nations, 1988.

**Table A-4.   Principal Causes of Death, Less-Developed Nations, 1980s**

| Nation and Year | Death Rate per 100,000 | Principal Causes of Death | Death Rate from Cause per 100,000 | Percentage of Total National Mortality from Cause |
|---|---|---|---|---|
| Brazil, 1982 | 592 | Cerebrovascular | 52 | 9 |
| | | Cancer | 51 | 9 |
| | | Ischemic heart disease | 45 | 8 |
| | | Other circulatory diseases | 42 | 7 |
| | | Perinatal mortality | 41 | 7 |
| | | Accidents | 34 | 6 |
| | | Ill-defined causes | 126 | 21 |
| Cape Verde, 1980 | 771 | Dysentery and gastroen-teritis | 95 | 12 |
| | | Ischemic heart disease | 64 | 8 |
| | | Other heart disease | 57 | 7 |
| | | Perinatal mortality | 49 | 6 |
| | | Cancer | 48 | 6 |
| | | Accidents | 26 | 3 |
| | | Ill-defined causes | 192 | 25 |
| Egypt, 1982 | 992 | Gastroenteritis | 146 | 15 |
| | | Other circulatory diseases | 113 | 11 |
| | | Perinatal mortality | 37 | 4 |
| | | Cancer | 18 | 2 |
| | | Ischemic heart disease | 16 | 2 |
| | | Accidents | 16 | 2 |
| | | Cerebrovascular | 12 | 1 |
| | | Ill-defined causes | 226 | 23 |
| Mexico, 1982 | 560 | Accidents | 72 | 13 |
| | | Cancer | 57 | 10 |
| | | Dysentery and gastroen-teritis | 47 | 8 |
| | | Other circulatory diseases | 42 | 8 |
| | | Perinatal mortality | 34 | 6 |
| | | Ischemic heart disease | 23 | 4 |
| | | Ill-defined causes | 30 | 4 |
| Peru | 469 | Accidents | 60 | 13 |
| | | Perinatal mortality | 44 | 9 |
| | | Gastroenteritis | 41 | 9 |
| | | Cancer | 33 | 7 |
| | | Ischemic heart disease | 14 | 3 |
| | | Cerebrovascular | 4 | 1 |
| | | Other circulatory diseases | 5 | 1 |
| | | Ill-defined causes | 35 | 7 |
| Philippines, 1981 | 599 | Influenza and pneumonia | 90 | 15 |
| | | Heart disease | 62 | 10 |
| | | Perinatal mortality | 56 | 9 |

(*continued*)

**Table A-4.** (*continued*)

| Nation and Year | Death Rate per 100,000 | Principal Causes of Death | Death Rate from Cause per 100,000 | Percentage of Total National Mortality from Cause |
|---|---|---|---|---|
| | | Tuberculosis | 53 | 9 |
| | | Dysentery and gastroen-teritis | 36 | 6 |
| | | Cancer | 31 | 5 |
| | | Cerebrovascular | 20 | 3 |
| | | Ill-defined causes | 54 | 9 |

*Source*: United Nations, 1988.

**Table A-5.  Life Expectancy by State and Sex, United States, 1979–1981**

| State | Life Expectancy at Birth | | Life Expectancy at Age 65 | |
|---|---|---|---|---|
| | Male | Female | Male | Female |
| Alabama | 68.3 | 76.8 | 13.7 | 18.2 |
| Alaska | 68.7 | 76.9 | 13.8 | 18.1 |
| Arizona | 70.5 | 78.3 | 15.1 | 19.2 |
| Arkansas | 69.7 | 77.8 | 14.4 | 18.6 |
| California | 71.1 | 78.0 | 14.7 | 18.7 |
| Colorado | 71.8 | 78.8 | 14.8 | 19.1 |
| Connecticut | 71.5 | 78.6 | 14.4 | 18.7 |
| Delaware | 69.6 | 76.8 | 13.5 | 18.0 |
| District of Columbia | 64.5 | 73.7 | 13.4 | 17.7 |
| Florida | 70.1 | 78.0 | 15.3 | 19.3 |
| Georgia | 68.0 | 76.4 | 13.5 | 18.1 |
| Hawaii | 74.1 | 80.3 | 16.6 | 20.1 |
| Idaho | 71.5 | 79.2 | 15.0 | 19.2 |
| Illinois | 69.6 | 77.1 | 13.9 | 18.1 |
| Indiana | 70.2 | 77.5 | 13.8 | 18.1 |
| Iowa | 72.0 | 79.6 | 14.7 | 19.4 |
| Kansas | 71.6 | 79.0 | 14.8 | 19.3 |
| Kentucky | 69.1 | 77.1 | 13.8 | 18.0 |
| Louisiana | 67.6 | 75.9 | 13.6 | 17.7 |
| Maine | 70.8 | 78.4 | 14.1 | 18.6 |
| Maryland | 69.7 | 76.8 | 13.6 | 17.9 |
| Massachusetts | 71.3 | 78.5 | 14.2 | 18.5 |
| Michigan | 70.1 | 77.3 | 13.9 | 18.2 |
| Minnesota | 72.5 | 79.8 | 15.0 | 19.5 |
| Mississippi | 67.6 | 76.4 | 13.9 | 18.1 |
| Missouri | 69.9 | 77.7 | 14.0 | 18.5 |
| Montana | 70.5 | 77.7 | 14.6 | 18.7 |
| Nebraska | 71.7 | 79.3 | 14.8 | 19.3 |
| Nevada | 69.3 | 76.5 | 14.1 | 18.1 |
| New Hampshire | 71.4 | 78.4 | 14.2 | 18.6 |
| New Jersey | 70.5 | 77.4 | 14.1 | 17.9 |
| New Mexico | 69.9 | 78.3 | 15.1 | 19.1 |
| New York | 70.0 | 77.2 | 14.1 | 18.1 |
| North Carolina | 68.6 | 77.3 | 13.8 | 18.5 |
| North Dakota | 72.1 | 79.7 | 15.2 | 19.4 |
| Ohio | 69.9 | 77.1 | 13.6 | 17.9 |
| Oklahoma | 69.6 | 77.8 | 14.2 | 18.8 |
| Oregon | 71.3 | 78.8 | 14.7 | 19.1 |
| Pennsylvania | 69.9 | 77.2 | 13.6 | 17.8 |
| Rhode Island | 71.0 | 78.3 | 14.1 | 18.6 |
| South Carolina | 67.6 | 76.1 | 13.5 | 17.9 |
| South Dakota | 71.0 | 79.2 | 14.9 | 19.6 |
| Tennessee | 69.2 | 77.5 | 14.0 | 18.5 |
| Texas | 69.7 | 77.7 | 14.3 | 18.6 |

(*continued*)

**Table A-5.**  (*continued*)

| State | Life Expectancy at Birth | | Life Expectancy at Age 65 | |
|---|---|---|---|---|
| | Male | Female | Male | Female |
| Utah | 72.4 | 79.2 | 15.1 | 19.0 |
| Vermont | 71.1 | 78.5 | 14.1 | 18.7 |
| Virginia | 69.6 | 77.3 | 13.6 | 18.1 |
| Washington | 71.7 | 78.6 | 14.6 | 18.9 |
| West Virginia | 68.9 | 76.9 | 13.7 | 18.0 |
| Wisconsin | 71.9 | 78.9 | 14.5 | 18.9 |
| Wyoming | 70.0 | 78.2 | 14.4 | 18.8 |
| Mean Life Expectancy in the United States, 1979–1981 | | | | |
| | 70.1 | 77.6 | 14.2 | 18.4 |

*Sources*: Metropolitan Life, 1986a, 1987b.

**Table A-6. Variations in Mortality Rates by States, Major Causes of Death**

| Disease (Period of Study) | Population | Range of Rates* (deaths/100,000 of population from cause) | U.S. Average Rate* | States in Ascending Order | | Source |
|---|---|---|---|---|---|---|
| | | | | Lowest Rates (three of each) | Highest Rates | |
| Cardiovascular Diseases (1985) | Men, 45+ | 735–1,269 | 1091 | HI, NM, AK | GA, SC, WV | 1 |
| | Women, 45+ | 457–735 | 657 | AK, HI, NM | WV, DC, LA | |
| Strokes (1985) | Both sexes, 45+ | 94–201 | | NM, DE, RI | GA, AL, SC | 2 |
| Influenza and Pneumonia (1979–1981) | Men, 45+ | 39–96 | 55 | RI, FL, NV | VA, MA, DC | 3 |
| | Women, 45+ | 19–38 | 30 | DE, FL, RI | CO, NY, MA | |
| Chronic Obstructive Pulmonary Disease (1986) | Both sexes | 17–49 | 30 | HI, DC, ND | CO, NV, WY | 4 |
| Diabetes Mellitus (1985) | Men, 45+ | 26–63 | 34 | OK, OR, AR | RI, DC, DE | 5 |
| | Women, 45+ | 22–57 | 33 | SD, OR, MN | MN, LA, DC | |
| Lung Cancer (1986) | Both sexes | 24–70 | 52 | UT, ND, HI | KY, NV, AL | 6 |
| Breast Cancer (1986) | Women | 23–41 | 33 | HI, ID, AR | NJ, RI, DE | 7 |
| Gastric Cancer (1979–1981) | Men, 45–84 | 15–44 | 21 | OK, KS, IA | NY, DC, HI | 8 |
| | Women, 45–84 | 6–24 | 9 | KS, WV, NV | NM, DC, HI | |

|  |  | Range | Rate | Lowest rates | Highest rates | Source |
|---|---|---|---|---|---|---|
| Cervical Cancer (1984–1986) | Women | 1.8–6.2 | 3.7 | UT, WY, MN | WV, SC, DC | 9 |
| Chronic Liver Disease and Cirrhosis (1980) | White Men, 35–74 | 15–60 | 37 | SD, ID, AK | NV, DC, CA | 10 |
|  | White Women, 35–74 | 7–37 | 17 | IA, AL, NE | HI, CA, NV |  |
| Motor Vehicle Fatalities (1979–1981) | White Men, 15–74 | 26–86 | 44 | RI, NJ, PA | NV, NM, WY | 11 |
|  | White Women, 15–74 | 9–28 | 14* | MA, NY, NJ | AZ, MT, NV |  |
| Homicide (1979–1981) | Men, 15–44 | 38–79 | 27 | ME, NH, MN | TX, LA, DC | 12 |
|  | Women, 15–44 | 2.1–14 | 6.2 | MN, IA, MA | AK, NV, DC |  |
| Suicide (1979–1981) | Men, 15–44 | 14–42 | 22 | NJ, DC, CT | CO, NM, NV | 13 |
|  | Women, 15–44 | 3–16 | 7 | NJ, NE, AL | AZ, WY, NV |  |
| Infant Mortality | Live births | 7–20/1,000 | 10 | WY, MT, NH | SC, AL, DC | 14 |

*Mortality rates adjusted for ages of U.S. population in 1940 except for infant mortality.

Sources: 1. Metropolitan Life, 1989b; 2. Metropolitan Life, 1989c; 3. Metropolitan Life, 1987c; 4. Centers for Disease Control, 1989d; 5. Metropolitan Life, 1989d; 6. Centers for Disease Control, 1989f; 8. Metropolitan Life, 1988a; 9. Centers for Disease Control, 1989g; 10. Metropolitan Life, 1989g; 10. Metropolitan Life, 1984; 11. Metropolitan Life, 1987d; 12. Metropolitan Life, 1987e; 13. Metropolitan Life, 1986c; 14. Metropolitan Life, 1988b.

# References

Altman, P. L. and Dittmer, P. S. (1972) Life spans: Animals. In *Biology Data Book*, Vol 1, pp. 229–235. Federation of American Societies for Experimental Biology, Bethesda, Maryland.

Ames, B. N. and Gold, L. S. (1991) Endogenous mutagens and the causes of aging and cancer. *Mutation Research* **250**, 3–16.

Anver, M. R., Cohen, B. J., Lattuada, C. P., and Foster, S. J. (1982) Age-associated lesions in barrier-reared male. Sprague-Dawley rats. *Experimental Aging Res.* **8**, 3–24.

Austad, S. N. and Fischer, K. E. (1991) Mammalian aging, metabolism, and ecology: Evidence from bats and marsupials. *Journal of Gerontology* **46**, B47–B53.

Ayanian, J. Z. and Epstein, A. M. (1991) Differences in the use of procedures between women and men hospitalized for coronary heart disease. *New England Journal of Medicine* **325**, 221–225.

Baba, N. X., Quattrochi, J. J., Baker, P. B., and Mueller, C. F. (1979) Cardiac and coronary pathology. In *Aging in Nonhuman Primates* (ed. D.M. Bowden), pp. 248–263. Van Nostrand Reinhold Company, New York.

Baker G. T., III and Sprott, R. L. (1988) Biomakers of aging. *Experimental Gerontology* **23**, 223–239.

Bank, L. and Jarvik, L. F. (1978) A longitudinal study of aging human twins. In *The Genetics of Aging* (ed. E. L. Schneider), pp. 303–333. Plenum Press, New York.

Baringa, M. (1991) How long is the human life span? *Science* **254**, 936–938.

Baringa, M. (1992) Novel function discovered for the cystic fibrosis gene. *Science* **256**, 444–445.

Baverstock, P. R., Adams, M., Polkinghorne, R. W., and Gelder, M. (1982) A sex-linked enzyme in birds—Z chromosome conservation but no gene dosage compensation. *Nature* **296**, 763–766.

Bell, C. A., Stout, N. A., Bender, T. R., Conroy, C. S., Crouse, W. E., and Myers, J. R. (1990) Fatal occupational injuries in the United States 1980–1985. *Journal of the American Medical Association* **263**, 3047–3050.

Berkel, J. and DeWaard, F. (1983) Mortality pattern and life expectancy of Seventh-Day Adventists in the Netherlands. *International Journal of Epidemiology* **12**, 455–459.

Berkman, L. F. (1988) The changing and heterogeneous nature of aging and longevity: A social and biomedical perspective. *Annual Review of Gerontology and Geriatrics* **8**, 37–68.

Bloom, B. R. and Murray, C. J. (1992) Tuberculosis: commentary on a reemergent killer. *Science* **257**, 1055–1064.

Blum, K., Noble, E. P., Sheridan, P. J., Montgomery, A., Richer, T., Jagadeswaran, P., Nogami, H., Briggs, A. H., and Lohn, J. B. (1990) Allelic association of human dopamine D2 receptor gene in alcoholism. *Journal of the American Medical Association* **263**, 2055–2060.

Blythe, R. (1969) *Akenfield: Portrait of an English Village*. Penguin Press, London.

Bolton, W. K., Benton, F. R., McClay, J. G., and Sturgill, B. C. (1976) Spontaneous glomerular sclerosis in aging Sprague-Dawlay rats. *American Journal of Pathology* **85**, 277–302.

Bowden, D. M. (1979) Aging research in nonhuman primates. In *Aging in Nonhuman Primates* (ed. D.M. Bowden), pp. 1–13. Van Nostrand Reinhold Company, New York.

Bowden, D. M. (1984) Aging. *Advances in Veternary Science and Comparative Medicine* **28**, 305–341.

Brandfonbrener, M., Landowne, M., and Shock, N. W. (1955) Changes in cardiac output with age. *Circulation* **12**, 557–566.

Bravo, R. R., Frank, R., Blundell, P. A., and MacDonald-Bravo, H. (1987) Cyclin/PCNA is the ancillary protein of DNA polymerase delta. *Nature* **326**, 515–527.

Brody, J. A. and Brock, D. B. (1985) Epidemiologic and statistical characteristics of the United States elderly population. In *Handbook of the Biology of Aging* (eds. C. E. Finch and E. L. Schneider), pp. 3–26. Van Nostrand Reinhold, New York.

Brown, G., Albers, J. J., Fisher, D. L., Schaefer, S. M., Lin, J-T., Kaplan, C., Zhao, X-Q, Bisson, B. D., Fitzpatrick, V. F., and Dodge, H. T. (1990) Regression of coronary artery disease as a result of intensive lipid-lowering therapy in men with high levels of apolipoprotein B. *New England Journal of Medicine* **323**, 1289–1298.

Buckley, R. H. (1986) Humoral immunodeficiency. *Clinical Immunology and Immunopathology* **40**, 13–24.

Bull, J. J. (1983) *Evolution of Sex Determining Mechanisms*. Benjamin Cummings Publishing Co., Menlo Park.

Bureau of Foreign and Domestic Commerce. (1914) *Statistical Abstract, 1913*. Government Printing Office, Washington, D.C.

Bureau of the Census. (1975) *Historical Statistics of the United States Colonial Times to 1970*. U.S. Department of Commerce, Washington, D.C.

Bureau of the Census. (1987) In *1980 Census of the Population* Vol. 1, Chapter B, Part 1. Department of Commerce, Washington, D.C.

Bureau of the Census. (1989) In *Statistical Abstract of the United States*. U.S. Department of Commerce, Washington, D.C.

Burgoyne, P. S. (1989) Thumbs down on zinc finger. *Nature* **342**, 860–862.

Burke, G. L., Sprafka, J. M., Folsom, A. R., Hahn, L. P., Luekper, R. V., and Blackburn, H. (1991) Trends in serum cholesterol levels from 1980 to 1987. *New England Journal of Medicine* **324**, 941–946.

Burns, A., Jacoby, R., Luthart, P., and Levy, R. (1990) Cause of death in Alzheimer's disease. *Age and Ageing* **19**, 241–244.

Busse, E. W. and Maddox, G. L. (1985) *The Duke Longitudinal Studies of Normal Aging, 1955–1980*. Springer Publishing Company, New York.

Callahan, D. (1987) *Setting Limits*. Simon and Schuster, New York.

Cameron, H. M. and McGoogan, E. (1981) A prospective study of 1152 hospital autopsies I. Inaccuracies in death certificates. *Journal of Pathology* **133**, 273–283.

Castelli, W. P. (1984) Epidemiology of coronary heart disease: The Framingham study. *American Journal of Medicine* (Suppl.) **76**, 4–12.

Cattanach, B. M. (1974) Position effect variegation in the mouse. *Genetical Research* **23**, 291–306.

Centers for Disease Control. (1989a) Summary of notifiable diseases, United States, 1988. *Morbidity and Morality Weekly Report* **37**, No. 54 (Suppl.)

Centers for Disease Control. (1989b) Update: Acquired immunodeficiency syndrome— United States 1981–1988. *Morbidity and Mortality Weekly Report* **38**, 229–236.

Centers for Disease Control. (1989c) Tobacco use by adults. *Morbidity and Mortality Weekly Report* **38**, 685–687.

Centers for Disease Control. (1989d) Chronic disease reports: Chronic obstructive pulmonary disease mortality—United States, 1986. *Morbidity and Mortality Weekly Report* **38**, 549–552.

Centers for Disease Control. (1989e) Chronic disease reports: Deaths from lung cancer— United States, 1986. *Morbidity and Mortality Weekly Report* **38**, 501–505.

Centers for Disease Control. (1989f) Chronic disease reports: Deaths from breast cancer among women—United States, 1986. *Morbidity and Mortality Weekly Report* **38**, 565–569.

Centers for Disease Control. (1989g) Chronic disease reports: Deaths from cervical cancer—United States 1984–1986. *Morbidity and Mortality Weekly Report* **38**, 650–654.

Centers for Disease Control. (1990) HIV prevalence estimates and AIDS case projections for the United States. *Mortality and Morbidity Weekly Report* **39**, No. RR16, 1–31.

Centers for Disease Control. (1991a) Cigarette smoking among adults—United States, 1988. *Mortality and Morbidity Report* **40**, 757–759, 765.

Centers for Disease Control. (1991b) Cigarette smoking among youth—United States 1989. *Mortality and Morbidity Weekly Report* **40**, 712–715.

Centers for Disease Control. (1991c) Smoking attributable mortality and years of potential life lost—United States, 1988. *Mortality and Morbidity Weekly Report* **40**, 62–63, 69–71.

Centers for Disease Control. (1992a) Cigarette smoking among adults—United States, 1990. *Mortality and Morbidity Weekly Report* **41**, 354–355, 361.

Centers for Disease Control. (1992b) Trends in alcohol-related traffic fatalities by sex—United States, 1982–1990. *Mortality and Morbidity Weekly Report* **41**, 195–197.

Cerami, A., Vlassara, H., and Brownlee, M. (1987) Glucose and Aging. *Scientific American* **256**,(6), 90–96.

Charlesworth, B. (1980) *Evolution in Age-Structured Populations*. Cambridge University Press, Cambridge.

Chiarelli, B. (1975) The study of primate chromosomes. In *Primate Functional Morphology and Evolution* (ed. R. H. Tuttle), pp. 103–128. Mouton Publishers, The Hague.

Ching, G. and Wang, E. (1990) Characterization of two populations of Statin and the relationship of their synthesis to the state of cell proliferation. *Journal of Cell Biology* **110**, 255–261.

Chu, S. Y., Buehler, J. W., and Berkelman, R. L. (1990) Impact of the human immunodeficiency virus epidemic on mortality in women of reproductive age—United States. *Journal of the American Medical Association* **264**, 225–229.

Cohen, B. (1964) Family patterns of mortality and life span. *Quarterly Review of Biology* **39**, 130–181.

Cohen, J. B. and Brody, J. A. (1981) The epidemiologic importance of psychosocial factors in longevity. *American Journal of Epidemiology* **114**, 451–461.

Coleman, G. L., Barthold, S. W., Osbaldeston, G. W., Foster, S. J., and Jonas, A. M. (1977) Pathological changes during aging in barrier-reared Fischer 344 male rats. *Journal of Gerontology* **32**, 258–278.

Colsher, P. L. and Wallace, R. N. (1989) Is modest alcohol consumption better than none at all? An epidemiologic assessment. *Annual Review of Public Health* **10**, 203–219.

Comfort, A. (1960) Longevity and mortality in dogs of four breeds. *Journal of Gerontology* **15**, 126–129.

Comfort, A. (1979) *The Biology of Senescence*. Elsevier, New York.

Committee on Animal Models for Research in Aging. (1981) *Mammalian Models for Research on Aging*. National Academy Press, Washington, D.C.

Coren, S. and Halpern, D. F. (1991) Left-handedness: A predictor for decreased fitness. *Psychological Bulletin* **109**, 90–106.

Cotran, R. S., Kumar, V., and Robbins, S. L. (1989) *Robbins Pathologic Basis of Disease*. W. B. Saunders, Philadelphia.

Cristofalo, V. J. (1988) An overview of the theories of biological aging. In *Emergent Theories of Aging* (eds. J. E. Birren and V. L. Bengtson), pp. 119–127. Springer, New York.

Cutler, R. G. (1975) Evolution of human longevity and the genetic complexity governing aging rate. *Proceedings of the National Academy of Science* **72**, 4664–4668.

Cutler, R. G. (1985) Dysdifferentiative hypothesis of aging: A review. In *Molecular Biology of Aging: Gene Stability and Gene Expression* (eds. R. S. Sohal, L. S. Birnbaum, and R. G. Cutler), pp. 307–340. Raven Press, New York.

Daniels, G. L. (1968) Ovulation and longevity of the Japanese quail (*Conturnix conturnix japonica*) under constant illumination. *Poultry Science* **47**, 1875–1878.

Deevey, E. S., Jr. (1947) Life tables for natural populations of animals. *Quarterly Review of Biology* **22**, 283–314.

Diamond, J. M. (1982) Big bang reproduction and aging in male marsupial mice. *Nature* **298**, 115–116.

Dilman, V. H. (1981) *The Law of Deviation of Homeostasis and Disease of Aging.* John Wright, PSG Inc. Boston.

Donato, H. and Sohal, R. S. (1981) Lipofuscin. In *Handbook of Biochemistry of Aging* (ed. J. R. Florini), pp. 221–227. CRC Press, Boca Raton, Florida.

Dublin, L. I. (1922) The possibility of extending human life. *The Harvey Lectures* **18**, 46–71.

Durand, J. D. (1960) Mortality estimates from Roman tombstone inscriptions. *American Journal of Sociology* **65**, 365–373.

Editorial. (1987) Made to last. *Lancet* **II**, 835–836.

Ehrhardt, A. A. and Meyer-Bahlburg, H.F.L. (1981) Effects of prenatal sex hormones on gender-related behavior. *Science* **211**, 1312–1318.

Eichner, E. R. (1985) Alcohol versus exercise for coronary protection. *American Journal of Medicine* **79**, 231–240.

Eisner, E. (1967) Actuarial data for the Bengalese finch (*Lonchura striata:* Fam. Estrildidae) in captivity. *Experimental Gerontology* **2**, 187–189.

Ershler, W. B., Moore, A. L., and Socinsky, M. H. (1985) Specific antibody synthesis *in vitro*. III. Correlation of *in vivo* and *in vitro* antibody response to influenza immunization in young and old subjects. *Journal of Clinical and Laboratory Immunology* **16**, 63–67.

Estivil, X., McLean, C., Nunes, V., Casals, T., Gallano, P., Scambler, P., and Williamson, R. (1989) Isolation of a new DNA marker in linkage disequilibrium with cystic fibrosis situated between J3.ll (D758) and IRP. *American Journal of Human Genetics* **44**, 704–710.

Evans, D. A., Funkenstein, H. H., Albert, M. S., Scherr, P. A., Cook, N. R., Chown, M. J., Hebert, L. E., Hennekens, C. H., and Taylor, J. O. (1989) Prevalence of Alzheimer's disease in a community population of older persons. *Journal of the American Medical Association* **262**, 2551–2556.

Faust, J. B. and Meeker, T. C. (1992) Amplification and expression of the bcl 1 in human solid tumor cell lines. *Cancer Research* **52**, 2460–2463.

Fearon, E. R., Winkelstein, J. A., Civin, C. I., Pardoll, D. M., and Vogelstein, B. (1987) Carrier detection in X-linked agammaglobulinemia by analysis of X-chromosome inactivation. *New England Journal of Medicine* **316**, 427–431.

Federman, D. D. (1987) Mapping the X-chromosome. *New England Journal of Medicine* **317**, 161–162.

Fesus, L., Davies, P. J., and Piacentini, M. (1991) Apoptosis: Molecular mechanisms in programmed cell death. *European Journal of Cell Biology* **55**, 170–177.

Fiennes, R. N. T.-W. ed. (1972) *Pathology of Simian Primates.* S. Karger, Basel.

Finch, C. E. (1987) Neural and endocrine determinants of senescence: Investigation of causality and reversibility by laboratory and clinical interventions. In *Modern Biological Theories of Aging* (eds. H. R. Warner, R. N. Butler, R. L. Sprott, and E. L. Schneider), pp. 261–308. Raven Press, New York.

Finch, C. E. (1990) *Longevity, Senescence, and the Genome*. University of Chicago Press, Chicago.

Food and Agriculture Organization. (1992) *World Food Supplies and Prevalence of Chronic Undernutrition in Developing Regions as Described in 1992*. Food and Agriculture Organization, Rome.

Foster, D., Klinger-Vartabidian, L., and Wispe, L. (1984) Male longevity and age differences between spouses. *Journal of Gerontology* **39**, 117–120.

Fraser, G. E. (1988) Determinants of ischemic heart disease in Seventh-day Adventists: A review. *American Journal of Clinical Nutrition* **48**, 833–836.

Frick, H. M. and others. (1987) Helsinki heart study: Primary prevention trial with gemfibrozil in middle-aged men with dyslipidemia. *New England Journal of Medicine* **317**, 1237–1245.

Friedberg, E. C. (1985) *DNA Repair*. W. H. Freeman, New York.

Friedman, D. B. and Johnson, T. E. (1988a) Three mutants that extend both mean and maximum life span of the nematode, Caenorhabditis elegans, define the age-1 gene. *Journal of Gerontology* **43**, B102–B109.

Friedman, D. B. and Johnson, T. E. (1988b) A mutation in the Age-1 gene in *Caenorhabditis elegans* lengthens life and reduces hermaphrodite fertility. *Genetics* **118**, 75–86.

Fries, B. (1983) Roman life expectancy: The Panonian evidence. *Phoenix* **37**, 328–344.

Fries, J. F. (1989) The compression of morbidity: Near or far? *Milbank Quarterly* **67**, 208–232.

Fries, J. F. (1990) The sunny side of aging. *Journal of the American Medical Association* **263**, 2354–2355.

Fries, J. F. and Crapo, L. M. (1981) *Vitality and Aging*. W. H. Freeman, New York.

Gartler, S. M. and Riggs, A. D. (1983) Mammalian X-chromosome inactivation. *Annual Review of Genetics* **17**, 155–190.

Gelman, R., Watson, A., Bronson, R., and Yunis, E. (1988) Murine chromosomal regions correlated with longevity. *Genetics* **118**, 693–704.

Gerschenson, I. F. and Rotello, R. J. (1992) *FASEB Journal* **6**, 2450–2455

Gilbert, C. (1967) When did a man in the Renaissance grow old? *Studies in the Renaissance* **14**, 7–32.

Gittings, R. (1968) *John Keats*. Little Brown and Company, Boston.

Gloth F. M., III. and Burtonk, J. R. (1990) Autopsies and death certificates in the chronic care setting. *Journal of the American Geriatric Society* **38**, 151–155.

Goldbourt, U. and Neufeld, H. N. (1986) Genetic aspects of atherosclerosis. *Atheroscloerosis* **6**, 357–377.

Goldman, L. and Cook, E. F. (1984) The decline in ischemic heart disease mortality rates. *Annals of Internal Medicine* **101**, 825–836.

Goodall, J. (1971) *In the Shadow of Man*. Houghton Mifflin Co., Boston.

Goodman, M. and Lasker, G. W. (1975) Molecular evidence as to man's place in nature. In *Primate Functional Morphology and Evolution* (ed. R. H. Tuttle), pp. 71–102. Mouton Publishers, The Hague.

Gordis, E., Tabokoff, B. Goldman, D., and Berg, K. (1990) Finding the gene(s) for alcoholism. *Journal of the American Medical Association* **263**, 2094–2095.

Graham, C. E., Kling, O. R., and Steiner, R. A. (1979) Reproductive senescence in female nonhuman primates. In *Aging in Nonhuman Primates* (ed. D. M. Bowden), pp. 183–202. Van Nostrand Reinhold Company, New York.

Gray, J. E., van Zwieten, M. J., and Hollander, C. F. (1982) Early light microscopic changes of chronic progressive nephrosis in several strains of aging laboratory rats. *Journal of Gerontology* **37**, 142–150.

Grundy, S. M. (1988) HMG-CoA reductase inhibitors for treatment of hyper-cholesterolemia. *New England Journal of Medicine* **319**, 24–33.

*Guinness Book of World Records*. Bantam Books, New York.

Guralnik, J. M. and Kaplan, G. A. (1989) Predictors of healthy aging: Prospective evidence from the Alameda County study. *American Journal of Public Health* **79**, 703–709.

Guralnik, J. M., Yanagashita, M., and Schneider, E. L. (1988) Projecting the older population of the United States: Lessons from the past and prospects for the future. *Milbank Quarterly* **66**, 283–308.

Hall, K. Y., Hart, R. W., Benirschke, K., and Walford, R. L. (1984) Correlation between ultra-violet induced DNA repair in primate lymphocytes and fibroblasts and species maximum achievable life span. *Mechanisms of Aging and Development* **24**, 153–173.

Halliwell, B., ed. (1987) *Oxygen Radicals and Tissue Injury*. Federation of American Scientists for Experimental Biology, Bethesda.

Hamilton, J. B. (1948) The role of testicular secretions as indicated by the effects of castration in man and by studies of pathological conditions and short lifespan associated with maleness. *Recent Progress in Hormone Research* **3**, 257–324.

Hansen, M. F. and Cavenee, W. K. (1987) Genetics of cancer predisposition. *Cancer Research* **47**, 5518–5527.

Hansen, M. H. (1986) *Demography and Democracy: The Number of Athenian Citizens in the Fourth Century B.C.* forlaget systime A/G, Copenhagen.

Harrison, D. E. and Archer, J. R. (1983) Physiological assays for biological age in mice: Relationship of collagen, renal function and longevity. *Experimental Aging Research* **9**, 245–251.

Harrison, D. E. and Archer, J. R. (1987) Genetic differences in effects of food restriction on aging in mice. *Journal of Nutrition* **117**, 376–382.

Harrison, D. E. and Archer, J. R. (1988) Editorial. Natural selection for extended longevity from food restriction. *Growth, Development and Aging* **52**, 65.

Harrison, D. E., Astle, C. M., and Lerner, C. (1984) Ultimate erythropoietic repopulating abilities of fetal, young, adult, and old adult cells compared using repeated irradiation. *Journal of Experimental Medicine* **160**, 759–771.

Hart, R. W. and Setlow, R. B. (1974) Correlation between deoxynucleic acid excision-repair and life-span in a number of mammalian species. *Proceedings of the National Academy of Science* **71**, 2169–2173.

Hart, R. W. and Turturro, A. (1987) Part I: Evolution of life span in placental mammals. In *Modern Biological Theories of Aging* (eds. H. R. Warner, R. N. Butler, R. W. Sprott, and E. L. Schneider), pp. 5–18, Raven Press, New York.

Hart, R. W., Sacher, G. A., and Hoskins, T. L. (1979) DNA repair in a short- and long-lived rodent species. *Journal of Gerontology* **34**, 808–817.

Hassold, T. H., Quillen, S. D., and Yamane, J. A. (1983) Sex ratio in spontaneous abortions. *Annals of Human Genetics* **47**, 39–47.

Haug, J. A., Høstmark, A. T., and Spydevold, O. (1984) Plasma lipoprotein responses to castration and androgen substitution in rats. *Metabolism* **33**, 465–470.

Hausman, P. B. and Weksler, M. E. (1985) Changes in the immune response with age. In *Handbook of the Biology of Aging* (eds. C. E. Finch and E. L. Schneider), pp. 414–432. Van Nostrand Reinhold, New York.

Hayflick, L. (1965) The limited *in vitro* lifetime of human diploid cell strains. *Experimental Cell Research* **37**, 614–636.

Hayflick, L. (1985) Theories of biological aging. *Experimental Gerontology* **20**, 145–159.

Hayflick, L. (1987) The human life-span. In *Realistic Expectations for Long Life* (ed. G. Lesnoff-Caravaglia), pp. 17–34. Human Sciences Press, New York.

Hayflick, L. and Moorhead, P. S. (1961) The serial cultivation of human diploid cell strains. *Experimental Cell Research* **25**, 585–621.

Hazzard, W. R. (1986) Biological basis of the sex differential in longevity. *Journal of the American Geriatrics Society* **34**, 455–471.

Hazzard, W. R. (1990) A central role of sex hormones in the sex differential in lipoprotein metabolism, atherosclerosis, and longevity. In *Gender, Health, and Longevity: Multidisciplinary Perspectives* (eds. M. G. Ory and H. R. Warner), pp. 87–108. Springer, New York.

Herrick, J. B. (1912) Clinical features of sudden obstruction of the coronary arteries. *Journal of the American Medical Association* **59**, 2015–2020.

Hoch, S. L. (1986) *Serfdom and Social Control in Russia: Petrovskoe, A Village in Tambov*. University of Chicago Press, Chicago.

Holden, C. (1983) Can smoking explain ultimate gender gap? *Science* **221**, 1034.

Holden, C. (1990) Primate secret to longevity. *Science* **250**, 1335.

Holden, C. (1991) Probing the complex genetics of alcoholism. *Science* **251**, 163–164.

Holehan, A. M. and Merry, B. J. (1986) The experimental manipulation of aging by diet. *Biological Reviews* **61**, 329–368.

Holliday, R. (1987a) The inheritance of epigenetic defects. *Science* **239**, 163–169.

Holliday, R. (1987b) X-chromosome reactivation. *Nature* **327**, 661–662.

Honig, G. R. and Adams J. G., III. (1986) *Human Hemoglobin Genetics*. Springer, New York.

Hopkins, K. (1966) On the probable age structures of the Roman population. *Population Studies* **20**, 245–264.

Hopkins, D. D., Grant-Worley, J. A., and Bollinger, T. L. (1989) Survey of cause-of-death query criteria used by state vital statistics programs in the US and the efficacy of the criteria used by the Oregon vital statistics program. *American Journal of Public Health* **79**, 570–574.

Horm, J. W. and Kessler, L. G. (1986) Falling rates of lung cancer in men in the U.S. *Lancet* **I**, 425–426.

Howell, T. H. (1988) Aristotle's remarks on old men. *Age and Ageing* **17**, 352–353.

Hrdy, S. B. (1981) "Nepotists" and "altruists": The behavior of old females among macaques and langur monkeys. In *Other Ways of Growing Old: Anthropological Perspectives* (eds. P. T. Amoss and S. Harrell), pp. 59–76. Stanford University Press, Stanford.

Ianuzzi, M. C., Dean, M., Drumm, M. L., Hidaka, N., Cole, J. L., Perry, A., Stewart, C., Gerrard, B., and Collins, F. S. (1989) Isolation of additional polymorphic clones from the cystic fibrosis region using jumping from D7S8. *American Journal of Human Genetics* **44**, 695–703.

Iozzo, R. V., Kushwaha, R. S., Wight, T. N., and Hazzard, W. R. (1982) Cellular and subcellular distribution of $^{125}$I-labeled very low density lipoproteins in the liver of normal and estrogen treated rabbits. *American Journal of Pathology* **107**, 6–15.

Ishii, T., Hosoda, Y., and Maeda, K. (1980) Cause of death in the extreme aged—A pathologic survey of 5106 elderly persons 80 years old and older. *Age and Aging* **9**, 81–89.

Israel, R. A., Rosenberg, H. M., and Curtin, L. B. (1986) Analytical potential for multiple cause-of-death data. *American Journal of Epidemiology* **124**, 161–179.

James, G., Patton, R. E., and Heslin, A. S. (1955) Autopsy and death certificates don't agree as to cause of death. *Public Health Reports* **70**, 39–51.

Johnson, T. E. (1988) Genetic specifications of life span: Processes, problems, and potentials. *Journal of Gerontology* **43**, B87–B92.

Johnson, T. E. (1990) *Caenorhabditis elegans* offers the potential for molecular dissection of the aging processes. In *Handbook of the Biology of Aging* (eds. E. L. Schneider and J. W. Rowe), pp. 45–62. Academic Press, New York.

Kane, J. P., Malloy, M. J., Tun, P., Phillips, N. R., and Havel, R. J. (1981) Normalization of low-density-lipoprotein levels in heterozygous familial hypercholesterolemia with a combined drug regimen. *New England Journal of Medicine* **304**, 251–258.

Kato, H., Harada, M., Tsuchiya, K., and Moriwaki, K. (1980) Absence of correlation between DNA repair in ultraviolet irradiated mammalian cells and life span of the donor species. *Japanese Journal of Genetics* **55**, 99–108.

Katz, S., Branch, L. G., Branson, M. H., Papsidero, J. A., Beck, J. C., and Greer, D. S. (1983) Active life expectancy. *New England Journal of Medicine* **309**, 1218–1224.

Kessler, M. J. and Rawlins, R. G. (1984) Absence of naturally acquired tetanus antitoxin in free-ranging Cayo Santiago rhesus monkeys (Macaca mulatta). *Journal of Medical Primatology* **13**, 353–357.

King, M. C. and Wilson, A. C. (1975) Evolution at two levels in humans and chimpanzees. *Science* **188**, 107–116.

Kircher, T. A., Nelson, J., and Burdo, H. (1985) The autopsy as a measure of accuracy of the death certificate. *New England Journal of Medicine* **313**, 1263–1269.

Kirkwood, T.B.L. (1985) Comparative and evolutionary aspects of longevity. In *Handbook of the Biology of Aging* (eds. C. E. Finch and E. L. Schneider), pp. 27–44. Van Nostrand Reinhold, New York.

Kirkwood, T.B.L. (1987) Immortality of the germ-line versus disposability of the soma.

In *Evolution of Longevity in Animals* (eds. A. D. Woodhead and K. H. Thompson), pp. 209–218. Plenum Press, New York.

Kirkwood, T.B.L. (1988) DNA, mutations and aging. *Mutation Research* **1**, 7–13.

Knodel, J. E. (1988) *Demographic Behavior of the Past*. Cambridge University Press, Cambridge.

Kohn, R. R. (1982) Cause of death in very old people. *Journal of the American Medical Association* **247**, 2793–2797.

Köhler, V. D. (1981) Lebensdauer Japanischer Wachteln bie Kafigemnzelhaltung Kurze Mitterlung. *Zeitschrift fur Versuchstierkunde* **2**, 239–241.

Kolonel, L. N. (1988) Variability in diet and its relation to risk in ethnic and migrant groups. In *Phenotypic Variation in Populations* (eds. A. D. Woodhead, M. A. Bender, and R. C. Leonard), pp. 129–136. Plenum Press, New York.

Koopman, P., Gubbay, J., Collingnon, J., and Lovell-Badge, R. (1989) Zfy gene expression patterns are not compatible with a primary role in mouse sex determination. *Nature* **342**, 940–942.

Kunkel, L. M., Smith, K. D., Boyer, S. H., Borgaonkar, D. S., Wachtel, S. S., Miller, O. J., Berg, W. R., Jones, H. W., and Rary, J. M. (1977) An analysis of human Y chromosome specific reiterated DNA in chromosome variants. *Proceedings of the National Academy of Science* **74**, 1245–1249.

Kuznetsova, S. (1987) Polymorphism of heterochromatin areas on chromosomes 1,9,16, and Y in long-lived subjects and persons of different ages in two regions of the Soviet Union. *Gerontology and Geriatrics* **6**, 177–186.

Laslett, P. (1985) Societal development and aging. In *Handbook of Aging and the Social Sciences* (eds. R. H. Binstock and E. Shanas), pp. 199–230. Van Nostrand Reinhold, New York.

Leaf, A. (1990) Long-lived populations (extreme old age). In *Principles of Geriatric Medicine and Gerontology* (eds. W. R. Hazzard, R. Andres, E. L. Bierman, and J. P. Blass), pp. 142–145. McGraw-Hill, New York.

Leckie, B. J. (1992) High blood pressure: Hunting the genes. *Bioessays* **14**, 37–41.

Lee, A. T. and Cerami, A. (1990) Modifications of proteins and nucleic acids by reducing sugars: Possible role in aging. In *Handbook of the Biology of Aging* (eds. E. L. Schneider and J. W. Rowe), pp. 116–130. Academic Press, New York.

Levi, W. M. (1953) *The Pigeon*. Levi Publishing Company, Sumter, South Carolina.

Levy, R. I. (1981) Declining mortality in coronary heart disease. *Arteriosclerosis* **1**, 312–325.

Li, F. P. (1988) Cancer families: Human models of susceptibility to neoplasia. *Cancer Research* **48**, 5381–5386.

Lieber, C. S. (1984) To drink (moderately) or not to drink. *New England Journal of Medicine* **310**, 846–848.

Lie, J. T. and Hammond, P. I. (1988) Pathology of the senescent heart: Anatomic observations on 237 autopsy studies of patients 90 to 105 years old. *Mayo Clinic Proceedings* **63**, 552–564.

Lindeman, R. C. (1981) The kidney. In *Handbook of Physiology in Aging* (ed. E. J. Masoro), pp. 175–187. CRC Press, Boca Raton, Florida.

Lipschitz, D. and Finch, C. A. (1985) The anemias. In *Principles of Geriatric Medicine* (eds. R. Andres, E. L. Bierman, and W. R. Hazzard), pp. 697–701. McGraw-Hill, New York.

Longino, C. F. (1988) Who are the oldest Americans? *The Gerontologist* **28**, 515–523.

Lopez, A. D. (1983) The sex mortality differential in developed countries. In *Sex Differentials in Mortality* (eds. A. D. Lopez and L. T. Ruzicka), pp. 53–120. Australian National University, Canberra.

Lopez, A. D. and Ruzicka, L. T., eds. (1983) *Sex Differentials in Mortality*. Australian National University, Canberra.

Luckinbill, L. S. and Clare, M. J. (1985) Selection for life span in *Drosophila melanogaster*. *Heredity* **55**, 9–18.

Lyon, J. L., Wetzler, H. P., Gardner, J. W., Klauber, M. R., and Williams, R. R. (1978) Cardiovascular mortality in Mormons and non-Mormons in Utah. *American Journal of Epidemiology* **108**, 357–366.

Lyon, J. L., Gardner, J. W., and West, D. W. (1988) Cancer risk and lifestyle: Cancer and Mormons from 1967–1975. In *Phenotypic Variations in Populations* (eds. A. D. Woodhead, M. A. Bender, and R. C. Leonard), pp. 137–161. Plenum Press, New York.

Lyon, M. F. (1972) X-chromosome inactivation and developmental patterns in mammals. *Biological Reviews* **47**, 1–35.

Maclusky, N. J. and Naftolin, F. (1981) Sexual differentiation in the central nervous system. *Science* **211**: 1294–1302.

Maeda, H., Gleiser, C. A., Masoro, E. J., Murata, I., McMahan, C. A., and Yu, B. P. (1985) Nutritional influences of aging of Fischer 344 rats: Pathology. *Journal of Gerontology* **40**, 671–708.

Makinodan, T. and Kay, M.M.B. (1980) Age influence on the immune system. *Advances in Immunology* **29**, 287–330.

Manton, K. G., and Soldo, B. J. (1985) Dynamics of health changes in the oldest old. *Milbank Quarterly* **63**, 206–285.

Manton, K. G. and Stallard, E. (1991) Cross-sectional estimates of active life expectancy for U.S. elderly and oldest old populations. *Journal of Gerontology* **46**, S170–S182.

Marshall, E. (1990) Experts clash over cancer data. *Science* **250**, 900–902.

Martin, G. M. (1977a) Cellular aging—Postreplicative cells. *American Journal of Pathology* **89**, 513–530.

Martin, G. M. (1977b) Cellular aging—Clonal senescence. *American Journal of Pathology* **89**, 484–511.

Martin, G. M. (1978) Genetic syndromes in man with potential relevance to the pathology of aging. In *Genetic Effects on Aging* (eds. D. Bergsma and D. E. Harrison), pp. 5–39. Alan R. Liss, New York.

Martin, G. M., Sprague, C. A., and Epstein, C. J. (1970) Replicative life-span of cultured human cells. Effects of donor's age, tissue, and genotype. *Laboratory Investigation* **23**, 86–92.

Mascart-Lemone, F., Delespasse, G., Servais, G., and Kunstler, M. (1982) Characterization of immunoregulatory T lymphocytes during aging by monoclonal antibodies. *Clinical and Experimental Immunology* **48**, 148–154.

Masoro, E. J. ed. (1981) *Handbook of Physiology in Aging*. CRC Press, Boca Raton, Florida.

Masoro, E. J. (1988) Minireview: Food restriction in rodents: An evaluation of its role in the study of aging. *Journal of Gerontology* **43**, B59–B64.

Masoro, E. J. (1990) Animal models in aging research. In *Handbook of the Biology of Aging* (eds. E. L. Schneider and J. W. Rowe), pp. 72–94. Academic Press, San Diego.

Mayr P. J. (1982) Evolutionary advantage of the menopause. *Human Ecology* **10**, 477–493.

Maxim, P. E. (1979) Social Behavior. In *Aging in Nonhuman Primates* (ed. D. M. Bowden), pp. 56–70. Van Nostrand-Reinhold, New York.

McClure, H. M. (1975a) Pathology of the Rhesus monkey. In *The Rhesus Monkey*, Vol. 2 (ed. G. H. Bourne), pp. 337–367. Academic Press, New York.

McClure, H. M. (1975b) Neoplasia in Rhesus monkeys. In *The Rhesus Monkey*, Vol. 2 (ed. G.H. Bourne), pp. 369–398. Academic Press, New York.

McKusick, V. A. (1975) *Mendelian Inheritance in Man*. Johns Hopkins University Press, Baltimore.

McKusick, V. A. (1988) *Mendelian Inheritance in Man*. Johns Hopkins University Press, Baltimore.

McKinlay, J. B. and McKinlay, S. M. (1977) The questionable contribution of medical measures to the decline of mortality in the United States in the twentieth century. *Milbank Memorial Fund Quarterly* **55**, 405–428.

McMillen, M. M. (1979) Differential mortality by sex in fetal and neonatal deaths. *Science* **204**, 89–91.

Meites, J., Goya, R., and Takahashi, S. (1987) Why the neuroendocrine system is important in aging processes. *Experimental Gerontology* **22**, 1–15.

Metropolitan Life. (1984) Regional variations in mortality from cirrhosis of the liver. *Statistical Bulletin* **65** (4), 22–28.

Metropolitan Life. (1986a) Longevity gains by state. *Statistical Bulletin* **67** (4), 12–17.

Metropolitan Life. (1986b) Suicide: An update. *Statistical Bulletin* **67** (2), 16–23.

Metropolitan Life. (1987a) Profile of centenarians. *Statistical Bulletin* **68** (1), 2–9.

Metropolitan Life. (1987b) Trends in longevity after age 65. *Statistical Bulletin* **68** (1), 10–17.

Metropolitan Life. (1987c) Pneumonia and influenza mortality on the increase. *Statistical Bulletin* **68** (2), 10–16.

Metropolitan Life. (1987d) Regional variations in mortality from motor vehicle accidents. *Statistical Bulletin* **68** (1), 26–31.

Metropolitan Life. (1987e) Homicide: A current overview. *Statistical Bulletin* **68** (4), 13–21.

Metropolitan Life. (1987f) Alcohol use in the United States. *Statistical Bulletin* **68** (1), 20–25.

Metropolitan Life. (1988a) Variations in mortality from gastric cancer. *Statistical Bulletin* **69** (1), 24–30.

Metropolitan Life. (1988b) Infant mortality, 1986. *Statistical Bulletin* **69** (2), 2–8.

Metropolitan Life. (1988c) Women's longevity advantage declines. *Statistical Bulletin* **69** (1), 18–23.

Metropolitan Life. (1989a) Life expectancy remains at record level. *Statistical Bulletin* **70** (3), 26–30.

Metropolitan Life. (1989b) Continued progress against cardiovascular diseases. *Statistical Bulletin* **70** (1), 16–23.

Metropolitan Life. (1989c) Progress against mortality from stroke. *Statistical Bulletin* **70** (2), 18–28.

Metropolitan Life. (1989d) Diabetes mortality update. *Statistical Bulletin* **70** (4), 24–34.

Metropolitan Life. (1989e) Hypertension in the United States: 1960 to 1980 and 1987 estimates. *Statistical Bulletin* **70** (2), 13–17.

Metropolitan Life. (1990) Major improvements in life expectancy: 1989. *Statistical Bulletin* **7** (3), 11–17.

Metropolitan Life. (1992) U.S. longevity at a standstill. *Statistical Bulletin* **72** (3), 2–9.

Migeon, B. R., Axelman, J., and Beggs, A. H. (1988) Effect of aging on reactivation of the human Z-linked HPRT locus. *Nature* **335**, 93–96.

Millar, W. J. (1983) Sex differentials in mortality by income level in urban Canada. *Canadian Journal of Public Health* **74**, 329–334.

Miller, R. A. (1990) Aging and the immune response. In *Handbook of the Biology of Aging* (eds. E. L. Schneider and J. W. Rowe), pp. 157–180. Academic Press, New York.

Miller, R. A. (1991) Accumulation of hyporesponsive calcium extruding memory T cells as a key feature of age-dependent immune dysfunction. *Clinical Immunology and Immunopathology* **58**, 305–317.

Miyamoto, M. M., Koop, B. H., Slightom, J. L., Goodman, M., and Tennant, M. R. (1988) Molecular systematics of higher primates: Genealogical relations and classification. *Proceedings of the National Academy of Science, USA* **85**, 7627–7631.

Montagu, A. (1952) *The Natural Superiority of Women*. Macmillan Co., New York.

Montagu, A. (1974) *The Natural Superiority of Women*. Collier Books, New York.

Moser, K. (1985) Levels and trends in child and adult mortality in Peru. *WFS Scientific Reports No. 27*. International Statistical Institute, Voorburg, Netherlands.

Munck, A., Guyre, R. M., and Holbrook, N. (1984) Physiological functions of glucocorticoids and their relation to pharmacological actions. *Endocrine Reviews* **5**, 25–44.

Murasko, D. M., Weiner, P., and Kaye, D. (1988) Association of lack of mitogen-induced lymphocyte proliferation with increased mortality in the elderly. *Aging, Immunology and Infectious Disease* **1**, 1–6.

Murphy, E. A. (1978) Genetics of longevity in man. In *The Genetics of Aging* (ed. E. L. Schneider), pp. 261–301. Plenum Press, New York.

Napier, J. R. and Napier, P. H. (1967) *A Handbook of Living Primates*. Academic Press, New York.

Nathanson, C. A. (1984) Sex differences in mortality. *Annual Review of Sociology* **10**, 191–213.

Nathanson, C. A. (1990) The gender–mortality ratio in developed countries: Demographic and sociocultural dimensions. In *Gender, Health, and Longevity: Multidisciplin-*

*ary Perspectives* (eds. M. G. Ory and H. R. Warner, pp. 3–24). Springer, New York.

National Center for Health Statistics. (1970) Mortality from selected causes by marital status. *Vital and Health Statistics* Series 20, No. 8, Parts A and B.

National Center for Health Statistics. (1965–1988) Editions of *Vital Statistics of the United States, 1965, 1966, 1967, etc.* (multiple volumes) U.S. Public Health Service, Washington.

National Center for Health Statistics. (1985) *U.S. Decennial Life Tables for 1979–81*. Department of Health and Human Services, publication 85-1150-1, Washington, D.C.

National Center for Health Statistics. (1988) *Vital Statistics of the United States, 1986*. U.S. Public Health Service, Washington.

National Center for Health Statistics. (1990) *Vital Statistics of the United States, 1987*. U.S. Public Health Service, Washington.

Neel, J. V. (1990) Toward an explanation of the human sex ratio. In *Gender, Health, and Longevity: Multidisciplinary Perspectives* (eds. M. G. Ory and H. R. Warner). pp. 57–72. Springer, New York.

Nielsen, J., Homma, A. and Byøin-Henriksen, T. (1977) Follow up 15 years after a geronto-psychiatric prevalence study: Conclusions concerning death, cause of death and life expectancy in relation to psychiatric diagnosis. *Journal of Gerontology* 32, 554–561.

Ning, Y. and Pereira-Smith, O. M. (1991) Molecular genetic approaches to the study of cellular senescence. *Mutation Research* 256, 303–310.

Nirenberg, T. D. and Miller, P. M. (1984) History and overview of the prevention of alcohol abuse. In *Prevention of Alcohol Abuse* (eds. P. M. Miller and T. D. Nirenberg), pp. 3–14. Plenum Press, New York.

Norwood, T. H., Smith, J. R., and Stein, G. H. (1990) Aging at the cellular level: The human fibroblast-like cell model. In *Handbook of the Biology of Aging* (eds. E. L. Schneider and J. W. Rowe), pp. 131–154. Academic Press, San Diego.

Novak, R., Bosze, A., Matkovics, B., and Fachet, J. (1979) Gene affecting superoxide dismutase activity linked to the histocompatibility complex in H-2 congenic mice. *Science* 207, 86–87.

Ohno, S. (1967) *Sex Chromosomes and Sex-linked Genes*. Springer, New York.

Olshansky, S. J. (1988) On forecasting mortality. *Milbank Quarterly* 66, 482–530.

Olshansky, S. J., Carnes, B. A., and Cassel, C. (1990) In search of Methuselah: Estimating the upper limits of human longevity. *Science* 250, 634–640.

Ose, L. and Tolleshaug, H. (1989) International symposium on familial hypercholesterolemia. *Arteriosclerosis* 9 (Suppl.) Il–I168.

Osler, W. (1901) *The Principles and Practice of Medicine*, fourth ed. D. Appleton and Company, New York.

Otten, M. W., Teutsch, S. M., Williamson, D. F., and Marks, J. P. (1990) The effect of known risk factors on the excess mortality of black adults in the United States. *Journal of the American Medical Association* 263, 845–850.

Paffenholz, V. (1978) Correlation between DNA repair of embryonic fibroblasts and different life spans of 3 inbred mouse strains. *Mechanisms of Aging and Development* 7, 131–150.

Palmer, M. S., Sinclair, A. H., Berta, P., Ellis, N. A., Goodfellow, P. N., Abbas, N. E., and Fellous, M. (1989) Genetic evidence that ZFY is not the testis-determining factor. *Nature* **342**, 937–939.

Palmore, E. B. (1982) Predictors of the longevity difference: A 25 year follow-up. *The Gerontologist* **22**, 513–518.

Passannante, M.R.C. and Nathanson, C. A. (1987) Women in the labor force: Are sex mortality ratios changing? *Journal of Occupational Medicine* **29**, 21–28.

Peterson, C., Seligman, M.E.P., and Vaillant, G. E. (1988) Pessimistic explanatory style as a risk factor for physical illness: A thirty-five year longitudinal study. *Journal of Personality and Social Psychology* **55**, 23–28.

Peto, S., Gray, R., Collins, R., Wheatley, K., Hennekens, C., Jansrozik, G., Warlos, C., Hafner, B., Thompson, C., Norton, S., Gilliland, J., and Doll, R. (1988) Randomized trial of prophylactic daily aspirin in British male doctors. *British Medical Journal* **296**, 313–316.

Phillips, R. L., Kuzma, J. W., Beeson, W. L., and Lotz, T. (1980) Influence of selection versus lifestyle on risk of fatal cancer and cardiovascular disease among Seventh-Day Adventists. *American Journal of Epidemiology* **112**, 296–314.

Preston, S. H., Keyfitz, N., and Schoen, R. (1972) *Causes of Death: Life Tables for National Populations*. Seminar Press, New York.

Price, W. H., Kitchin, A. H., Burgon, P.R.S., Morris, S. W., Wenham, P. R., and Donald, P. M. (1989) DNA restriction fragment length polymorphisms as markers of familial coronary heart disease. *Lancet* **I**, 1407–1410.

Promislow, E. L. and Harvey, P. H. (1990) Living fast and dying young: A comparative analysis of life-history variation among mammals. *Journal of Zoology* **220**, 417–437.

Prothero, J. and Jürgens, K. D. (1987) Scaling of maximal lifespan in mammals: A review. In *Evolution of Longevity in Animals* (eds. A. D. Woodhead and K. H. Thompson), pp. 49–74. Plenum Press, New York.

Puxty, J.A.H., Fox, R. A., and Horan, M. A. (1983) Necropsies in the elderly. *Lancet* **I**, 1262–1264.

Rajput-Williams, J., Wallis, S. C., Yarnell, J., Bell, G. I., Knott, T. J., Sweetnam, P., Cox, N., Miller, N. E., and Scott, J. (1988) Variation in the apolipoprotein-B gene is associated with obesity, high blood cholesterol levels and increased risk of coronary heart disease. *Lancet* **II**, 1442–1445.

Remington, P. L., Novotny, T. E., Williamson, D. F., and Anda, R. F. (1989) State-specific progress toward the 1990 objective for the nation' for cigarette smoking prevalence. *American Journal of Public Health* **79**, 1416–1419.

Ricklefs, R. E. (1973) Fecundity, mortality, and avian demography. In *Breeding Biology of Birds* (ed. P. S. Farner), pp. 366–435. National Academy of Sciences, Washington.

Roberts-Thomson, I. C., Whittingham, S., Youngchaiyud, U., and Mackay, I. R. (1974) Aging, immune response, and mortality. *Lancet* **II**, 368–370.

Rodeheffer, R. J., Gerstenblith, G., Becker, L. C., Fleg, J. L., Weisfeldt, M. L., and Lakatta, E. G. (1984) Exercise cardiac output is maintained with advancing age in heathy human subjects: Cardiac dilation and increased stroke volume compensate for a diminished heart rate. *Circulation* **69**, 203–213.

Rodenhuis, S. and Slebos, R. J. (1992) Clinical significance of Ras oncogene activation in human lung cancer. *Cancer Research* **52** (Supplement), 2665S–2669S.

Rodin, J. (1986) Aging and health: Effects of the sense of control. *Science* **233**, 1271–1276.

Rogers, R. C. and Wofford, S. (1989) Life expectancy in less developed countries: Socioeconomic development or public health? *Journal of Biosocial Science* **21**, 245–252.

Rose, M. R. (1991) *Evolutionary Biology of Aging*. Oxford University Press, New York and Oxford.

Rose, M. R. and Graves, J. L., Jr. (1989) What evolutionary biology can do for gerontology. *Journal of Gerontology* **44**, B27–B29.

Rose, M. R., Dorey, M. L., Coyle, A. M., and Service, P. M. (1984) The morphology of postponed senescence in *Drosphila melanogaster. Canadian Journal of Zoology* **62**, 1576–1580.

Rosenwaike, I. (1985) *The Extreme Aged in America*. Greenwood Press, Westport, Connecticut.

Rowe, J. W. and Kahn, R. L. (1987) Human aging: Usual and successful. *Science* **237**, 143–149.

Rubin, R. T., Reinisch, J. M., and Haskett, R. F. (1981) Postnatal gonadal steroid effects on human behavior. *Science* **211**, 1318–1324.

Rudman, D., Feller, A. G., Nagraj, H. S., Gergans, G. A., Lalitha, P. Y., Goldberg, A. F., Schlenker, R. A., Cohn, L., Rudman, I. W., and Mattson, D. E. (1990) Effects of human growth hormone in men over 60 years old. *New England Journal of Medicine* **323**, 1–6.

Russell, J. C. (1987) *Medieval Demography*. AMS Press, New York.

Sacher, G. A. (1975) Maturation and longevity in relation to cranial capacity in hominid evolution. In *Primate Functional Morphology and Evolution* (ed. R. H. Tuttle), pp. 417–441. Mouton Publishers, The Hague.

Sacher, G. A. (1978) Evolution of longevity and survival characteristics in mammals. In *Genetics of Aging* (ed. E. L. Schneider), pp. 151–168). Plenum Press, New York.

Sacher, G. A. and Hart, R. W. (1978) Longevity, aging, and comparative cell and molecular biology of the house mouse, *Mus musculus,* and the white footed mouse, *Perromyscus leucopus.* In *Genetic Effects on Aging* (eds. D. Bergsma and D. E. Harrison), pp. 71–96. Alan R. Liss Inc., New York.

Sadik, N. (1989) *The State of World Population 1989*. United Nations Population Fund, New York.

Sager, R. (1989) Tumor suppressor genes: The puzzle and the promise. *Science* **246**, 1406–1411.

Sandberg, A. A., ed. (1983) *Cytogenetics of the Mammalian X-chromosome*. Alan R. Liss, New York.

Sandberg, A. A., ed. (1985) *The Y Chromosome*. Alan R. Liss, New York.

Schmidt, R. M. (1989) Healthy aging: Individual health trend assessment and intervention in the routine clinical practice. *The Gerontologist* **29**, special issue, 1A.

Schneider, E. L. and Reed, J. D. (1985) Life extension. *New England Journal of Medicine* **312**, 1159–1168.

Schneider, E. L. and Guralnik, J. (1990) The aging of America: Impact on health care costs. *Journal of the American Medical Association* **263**, 2335–2340.

Schoenborn, C. A. and Cohen, B. H. (1986) Trends in smoking, alcohol consumption, and other health practices among U.S. adults, 1977 and 1983. *Advance Data From Vital and Health Statistics of the National Center for Health Statistics, No. 118.* Department of Health and Human Service Publication PHS 86–1250.

Schultz, A. H. (1968) The recent hominid primates. In *Perspectives on Human Evolution* (eds. S. L. Washburn and P. C. Jay), pp. 122–195. Holt, Rinehart and Winston, New York.

Segal, P., Rifkind, B. M., and Shull, W. J. (1982) Genetic factors in lipoprotein variation. *Epidemiological Reviews* **4**, 137–160.

Shimada, F., Taira, M., Suzuki, Y., Hashimoto, N., Nozaki, D., Taira, M., Tatilana, M., Ebina, Y., Tawata, M., Onaya, T., Makino, H., and Yoshida, S. (1990) Insulin-resistant diabetes associated with partial deletion of insulin-receptor gene. *Lancet* **335**, 1179–1181.

Shiveley, C. and Mitchell, G. (1986a) Prenatal behavior in prosimian primates. In *Comparative Primate Biology* Vol. 2, Part A (eds. G. Mitchell and J. Erwin), pp. 217–243. Alan R. Liss, Inc. New York.

Shively, C. and Mitchell, G. (1986b) Perinatal behavior of anthropoid primates. In *Comparative Primate Biology* Vol. 2, Part A (eds. G. Mitchell and J. Erwin), pp. 245–294. Alan R. Liss, Inc. New York.

Shock, N. W. (1961) Physiological aspects of aging in man. *Annual Review of Physiology* **23**, 97–122.

Shock, N. W. (1984) *Normal Human Aging.* U.S. Department of Health and Human Services (NIH Publication No. 84–2450), Washington.

Simons, E. L. (1968) New fossil primates: A review. In *Perspectives on Human Evolution* (eds. S. L. Washburn and P. C. Jay), pp. 41–60. Holt, Rinehart, and Winston, New York.

Simons, E. L. (1989) Human origins. *Science* **245**, 1343–1350.

Smith, D.W.E. (1989) Is greater female longevity a general finding among animals? *Biological Reviews* **64**, 1–12.

Smith, D.W.E. and Warner, H. R. (1989) Does genotypic sex have a direct effect on longevity? *Experimental Gerontology* **24**, 277–288.

Smith, D.W.E. and Warner, H. R. (1990) Overview of biomedical perspectives: Possible relationships between genes on the sex chromosomes and longevity. In *Gender, Health, and Longevity: Multidisciplinary Perspectives* (eds. M. G. Ory and H. R. Warner), pp. 41–56. Springer, New York.

Smith, G. S. and Walford, R. L. (1977) Influence of the main histocompatibility complex on aging in mice. *Nature* **270**, 727–729.

Smith, S. M., Hoy, W. E., and Cobb, L. (1989) Low incidence of glomerulosclerosis in normal kidneys. *Archives of Pathology and Laboratory Medicine* **113**, 1253–1255.

Smith-Sonneborn, J. (1987) Longevity in the protozoa. In *Evolution of Longevity in Animals* (eds. A. D. Woodhead and K. H. Thompson), pp. 101–109. Plenum Press, New York.

Soldo, B. J. and Manton, K. G. (1985) Health status and service needs of the oldest old: Current patterns and future trends. *Milbank Quarterly* **63**, 286–318.

Sorensen, T.I.A., Nielsen, G. G., Andersen, P. K., and Teasdale, T. W. (1988) Genetic and environmental influences on premature death in adult adoptees. *New England Journal of Medicine* **318**, 727–732.

Sorlie, P., Rogot, E., Anderson, R., Johnson, N. J., and Backlund, E. (1992) Black–white mortality by differences in family income. *Lancet* **340**, 346–350.

Stadtman, E. R. (1988) Protein modification in aging. *Journal of Gerontology* **43**, B112–B120.

Stead, W. W., Senner, J. W., Reddick, W. T., and Lofgren, J. P. (1990) Racial differences in susceptibility to infection by *Mycobacterium tuberculosis*. *New England Journal of Medicine* **322**, 422–427.

Steering Committee of the Physicians' Health Study Research Group. (1989) Final report on the aspirin component of the ongoing physicians' health study. *New England Journal of Medicine* **321**, 129–135.

Steingart, R. M. and many co-authors. (1991) Sex differences in the management of coronary heart disease. *New England Journal of Medicine* **325**, 226–230.

Stephan, H., Baron, G., and Frahm, H. D. (1988) Comparative size of brains and brain components. In *Comparative Primate Biology* Vol. 4 (eds. H. D. Steklis and J. Erwin), pp. 1–38. Alan R. Liss, Inc. New York.

Stout, J. T. and Caskey, C. T. (1985) HPRT: Gene structure, expression, and mutation. *Annual Review of Genetics* **19**, 127–148.

Stringer, C. B. and Andrews, P. (1988) Genetic and fossil evidence for the origin of modern humans. *Science* **239**, 1263–1268.

Svanborg, A., Shibata, H., Hatano, S., and Matsuzaki, T. (1985) Comparison of ecology, ageing and state of health in Japan and Sweden, the present and previous leaders in longevity. *Acta Medica Scandinavica* **218**, 5–17.

Takagi, N. and Sasaki, M. (1974) A phylogenetic study of bird karryotypes. *Chromosoma* **46**, 91–120.

Takata, H., Ishii, T., Suzuki, M., and Sikiguchi, S. (1987) Influence of major genes on human longevity among Okinawan-Japanese centenarians and nonagenarians. *Lancet* **II**, 824–826.

Talal, N. (1981) Sex steroid hormones and systemic lupus erythematosis. *Arthritis and Rheumatism* **24**, 1054–1056.

Thomson, G. (1988) HLA disease associations: Models for insulin dependent diabetes mellitus and the study of complex human genetic disorders. *Annual Review of Genetics* **22**, 31–50.

Tice, R. R. and Setlow, R. B. (1985) DNA repair and replication in aging organisms and cells. In *Handbook of the Biology of Aging* (eds. C. E. Finch and E. L. Schneider), pp. 173–224. Van Nostrand Reinhold, New York.

Timaeus, J. (1984) Mortality in Lesotho: A study of levels, trends, and differentials based on retrospective survey data. *WFS Scientific Reports No. 59*. International Statistical Institute, Voorburg, Netherlands.

Tiwari, J. L. and Terasaki, P. I. (1985) *HLA and Disease Associations*. Springer-Verlag, Berlin.

Tolmasoff, J. M., Ono, T., and Cutler, R. G. (1980) Superoxide dismutase: Correlation with life-span and specific metabolic rate in primate species. *Proceedings of the National Academy of Science* **77**, 2777–2781.

Torrey, B. B., Kinsella, K., and Taeuber, C. M. (1987) *An Aging World*. Bureau of the Census, U.S. Department of Commerce, Washington.

Ullrich, S. J., Anderson, C. W., Mercer, W. E., and Appella, E. (1992) The p53 tumor suppressor protein, a modulator of cell proliferation. *Journal of Biological Chemistry* **267**, 15259–15262.

United Nations. (1979) *Demographic Yearbook, 1979*. United Nations, Department of International Economics and Social Affairs, Statistical Office, New York.

United Nations. (1988) *Demographic Yearbook, 1986*. United Nations, Department of International Economics and Social Affairs, Statistical Office, New York.

United Nations. (1990) *Demographic Yearbook, 1988*. United Nations, Department of International Economics and Social Affairs, Statistical Office, New York.

Vallois, H. V. (1961) The social life of early man: The evidence of skeletons. In *Social Life of Early Man* (ed. S. L. Washburn), pp. 214–235. Aldine Publishing Co., Chicago.

Van Poppel, F.W.A. (1981) Regional mortality differences in Western Europe: Review of the situation in the seventies. *Social Science and Medicine* **15D**, 341–352.

Vaupel, J. W. and Gowan, A. E. (1986) Passage to Methuselah: Some demographic consequences of continued progress against mortality. *American Journal of Public Health* **76**, 430–433.

Verbrugge, L. M. (1983) Women and men: Mortality and health of older people. In *Aging in Society: Selected Reviews of Recent Research* (eds. M. W. Riley, B. B. Hess, and K. Bond), pp. 139–173. Lawrence Erlbaum Associates, New Jersey.

Verbrugge, L. M. (1985) Gender and health: An update on hypotheses and evidence. *Journal of Health and Social Behavior* **26**, 146–182.

Verbrugge, L. M. and Madans, J. H. (1985) Social roles and health trends of American women. *Milbank Quarterly* **63**, 691–735.

Verbrugge, L. M. and Wingard, D. L. (1987) Sex differentials in health and mortality. *Women and Health* **12**, 103–143.

Vesselinovitch, D. (1988) Animal models and the study of atherosclerosis. *Archives of Pathology and Laboratory Medicine* **112**, 1011–1017.

Vigilant, L., Stoneking, M., Harpending, H., Hawkes, K., and Wilson, A. C. (1991) African populations and the evolution of human mitochondrial DNA. *Science* **253**, 1503–1508.

Vinovskis, M. A. (1971) The 1789 life table of Edward Wigglesworth. *Journal of Economic History* **31**, 570–590.

Wade, A. (1989) *Actuarial Studies: Social Security Area Population Projection 1989*. U.S. Department of Health and Human Services, Social Security Administration, Office of the Actuary, SSA Publication No. 11-11552, Washington.

Waldman, T. A. (1986) Immunodeficiency: Immunoregulation and immunogenetics. *Clinical Immunology and Immunopathology* **40**, 25–36.

Waldron, I. (1976) Why do women live longer than men. *Social Science and Medicine* **10**, 349–362.

Waldron, I. (1983) Sex differences in human mortality: The role of genetic factors. *Social Science and Medicine* **17**, 321–333.

Waldron, I. (1986) The contribution of smoking to sex differences in longevity. *Public Health Reports* **101**, 163–173.

Waldron, I. and Jacobs, J. A. (1988) Effects of labor force participation on women's health: Evidence from a longitudinal study. *Journal of Occupational Medicine* **30**, 977–984.

Walford, R. L., Jawaid, S., and Nalim, F. (1981) Evidence for *in vitro.* senescence of T-lymphocytes cultured from normal human peripheral blood. *Age* **4**, 67–70.

Waller, B. F. and Roberts, W. C. (1983) Cardiovascular disease in the very elderly: Analysis of 40 necropsy patients aged 90 years and over. *American Journal of Cardiology* **51**, 403–421.

Wareham, K. A., Lyon, M. F., Glenister, P. H., and Williams, E. D. (1987) Age related reactivation of an X-linked gene. *Nature* **327**, 725–727.

Weidenrich, F. (1939) The duration of life in fossil man in China and the pathological lesions found in the skeleton. *Chinese Medical Journal* **55**, 34–44.

Weisburger, J. H. (1991) Carcinogenesis in our food and cancer prevention. *Advances in Experimental Medicine and Biology* **289**, 137–151.

Weksler, M. E. (1990) A possible role for the immune system in the gender longevity differential. In *Gender, Health and Longevity: Multidisciplinary Perspective* (eds. M. G. Ory and H. R. Warner), pp. 109–118. Springer, New York.

Whitfield, J. E. (1992) Calcium signals and cancer. *Critical Reviews in Oncogenesis* **3**, 55–90.

Williams, A. F. and Lund, A. K. (1986) Seat belt use laws and occupant crash protection. *American Journal of Public Health* **76**, 1438–1442.

Wilson, J. D., Braunwald, E., Isselbacher, K. J., Petersdorf, R. G., Martin, J. B., Fauci, A. J., and Root, R. K. (1991) *Harrison's Principles of Internal Medicine*. McGraw-Hill, New York.

Wingard, D. L. (1984) The sex differential in morbidity, mortality, and lifestyle. *Annual Review of Public Health* **5**, 433–458.

Wolf, N. S., Giddens, W. E., and Martin, G. M. (1988) Life table analysis and pathologic observations in male mice of a long-lived hybrid strain (Af X C57B/6)F1. *Journal of Gerontology* **43**, 871–878.

Woodhead, A. D. (1978) Fish studies of aging. *Experimental Gerontology* **13**, 125–140.

World Health Organization. (1967) *The International Classification of Disease*, eighth revision. WHO Publications Centre, Geneva.

World Health Organization. (1977) *Manual of the Statistical Classification of Diseases*, ninth revision. United Nations, Geneva.

Yano, K., Reed, D. M., and McGee, D. L. (1984) Ten-year incidence of coronary heart disease in the Honolulu Heart Program. *American Journal of Epidemiology* **119**, 653–666.

Yu, B. P., Masoro, E. J., and McMahan, C. A. (1985) Nutritional influences on aging of Fischer 344 rats: I. Physical, metabolic and longevity characteristics. *Journal of Gerontology* **40**, 657–670.

Yunis, J. J. and Prakash, O. (1982) The origin of man: A chromosomal pictorial legacy. *Science* **215**, 1525–1529.

Zeman, F. D. (1942) Old age in ancient Egypt. *Journal of the Mount Sinai Hospital* **8**, 1161–1165.

# Index